On being in charge

A GUIDE TO MANAGEMENT IN PRIMARY HEALTH CARE

by

Rosemary McMahon, Elizabeth Barton & Maurice Piot

in collaboration with
Naomi Gelina & Felton Ross

Second edition

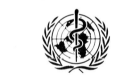

World Health Organization
Geneva
1992

WHO Library Cataloguing in Publication Data

McMahon, Rosemary

    On being in charge: a guide to management in primary health care/ by Rosemary
McMahon, Elizabeth Barton & Maurice Piot; in collaboration with Naomi Gelina &
Felton Ross. — 2nd ed.

    1.Primary health care — organization & administration — programmed texts I.Barton,
Elizabeth II.Piot, Maurice III.Title

    ISBN 92 4 154426 0   (NLM Classification: W 18)

TYPESET IN INDIA
PRINTED IN ENGLAND
89/B317 – Macmillan/Clays – 15,000

Contents

Acknowledgements

The following have participated in the team-work for the preparation of this revised edition of *On being in charge*, coordinated by, and under the responsibility of, Dr D. Flahault:

Dr F. Canonne, Dr J. Gallagher, and Mrs S. Dumont.

The authors are indebted to Dr J. Gallagher for Section 3.6, Chapter 3, Part II and for extensive assistance in editing this book, and to Dr D. Morley for Section 4.1, Chapter 4, Part III.

Others who kindly provided comments were:

Dr A. d'Almeida (Togo), Mr B. Benyounes (Morocco), Mr M. Gebrie (Ethiopia), Mrs H. Grandguillot (Médecins sans Frontières, France), Mrs N. Hamunen (Finland), Dr S. Moday (Turkey), Dr E. Mutabaruka (Rwanda) and Dr E. Parry (United Kingdom).

Introduction

The first edition of this book was prepared soon after the historic Conference of Alma-Ata and the adoption by the Member States of the World Health Organization of the goal of health for all by the year 2000 by means of primary health care. It has been used extensively throughout much of the world during a period when many health care systems have taken new directions as countries have begun to implement their strategies to attain this goal. WHO is acutely aware of the difficulties that must be overcome if countries are to transform the principles upon which there appears to be universal agreement into functioning health systems based on primary health care, and ultimately into credible or genuine states of health for all.

From an early stage in the movement to establish primary health care as the basis for achieving health for all, it was evident that the principal obstacle was weak management, particularly at the district level of health systems. There are many reasons for this. Primary health care is a complex concept requiring the most efficient use of resources, which are almost always scarce, and implying choice and the setting of priorities. It involves communities in making decisions about their own health care and in accepting responsibility for protecting their own health. In dealing with malnutrition or ensuring a safe water supply, for instance, it involves sectors other than the health sector. Generally it requires the best use to be made of various categories of health worker, many of whom may be inadequately trained for the work they are expected to do, unused to working in teams, or dissatisfied with their working conditions. Health care is often a matter of persuading or educating people to change certain kinds of behaviour that affect their health. Sometimes community health workers are so much part of their communities that they need continuous training and support to enable them to take a lead in matters of health.

There are so many different variables to consider and coordinate that the management of health services and health personnel is difficult and can never be perfect. However, the principles of health work are clear: the connection between the cause and the disease or disability must be broken. People can be educated and helped to work together to make a healthy environment. They can be helped to learn to behave in ways that will protect their own and their children's health, and thus avoid many of the causes of disease. However, they must be treated and cared for when they become ill.

Sometimes, the obstacles to good community health care services are so great that health workers seem to take refuge in doing what they can easily do, or what people expect of them, and simply stay in their health centres to treat those who come with symptoms of disease, without reference to cause. The patients return to the conditions that caused the disease and become ill again, and the health workers then miss the satisfaction of cooperating successfully with the people to make a healthy environment. Management is a systematic way of bringing about such cooperation. Its principles and methods are the same whether resources are plentiful or scarce, or conditions favourable or unfavourable. When resources are scarce and conditions are difficult the management effort necessary can also be difficult. Good management perseveres, however, and never loses sight of basic principles.

This guide to management is designed to help health managers — and nearly all health workers are managers in one way or another — to master by constant use the principles of good management.

Management principles are applied at all levels of a health care system — at the central or national level, in ministries of health and other national organizations and institutions; at the intermediate level, in regions or provinces or the states of a federal system, which may include ministries or other state authorities and tertiary- or secondary-level hospitals and health centres; and at district level, with its health centres and smaller units and district hospitals. The emphasis in this guide is on the district level, where high standards of management are vital to the functioning of health systems based on primary health care.

The district level

The form of organization of district health services based on primary health care obviously varies from country to country, but its essential characteristics are constant: full and universal accessibility, emphasis on promotion of health and prevention of disease and disability, intersectoral action, community involvement, and decentralization and coordination of all health services or systems, governmental and nongovernmental.

In a given country, a district is an organized unit of local government, and a district health subsystem is a more or less self-contained segment of the national health system. It comprises, first and foremost, a well defined population living within a clearly delineated administrative and geographic area, either urban or rural. It includes all individuals, institutions and sectors whose activities contribute to the improvement of health. It also includes self-care, all health staff and facilities up to and including the hospital at the first referral level, and logistic support services.

Health services and health teams

The relationship between various health personnel at different levels of the health care system is generally interpreted within the framework of an organization's hierarchical structure, as represented, for example, in the form of a pyramid.

Such a structure suggests a two-way relationship, between a superior and a subordinate: supervision becomes merged with direction. In many countries, health services, and more specifically primary health care services, at district level have adopted the functional concept of health teams. Those who make up the teams may belong to one level or more of the health system.

It is a common mistake to regard management as a function of those at the top of the pyramid only and to give it little attention at intermediate and district levels. The effect is that well conceived programmes fail because of confusion at the lower levels of the pyramid.

Good management is to organization what health is to the body — the smooth functioning of all its parts. It highlights priorities, adapts services to needs and changing situations, makes the most of limited resources, improves the standard and quality of services, and maintains high staff morale.

The management of a health centre includes the management of the health of the entire population it serves. When the health centre is well managed, the community is healthier. If the community's health is poor or not

Pyramid of health services

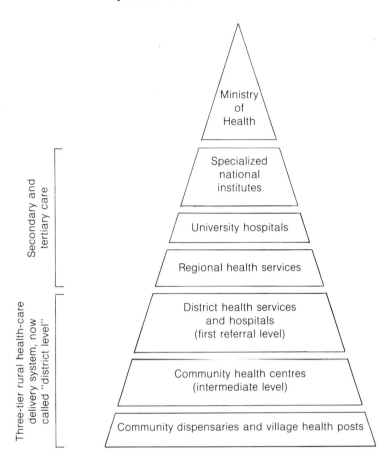

improving, it is likely that the health centre, and the community health services in general, are poorly managed. If the community's health is improving, good management ensures that the improvement is shared by everyone, young and old, poor and less poor, poorly educated and well educated.

How to use this guide

Those people who have used the earlier edition of this guide have found that it may be used in several ways:

A student who has so far learned only to care for patients in hospital is deprived for the first time, perhaps during a rural assignment, of the familiar technical and educational support available in a teaching hospital. Such a student could be advised to study first Parts II and IV and do the related exercises, and then to study Parts I and III.

This sequence would allow the student to begin to work on familiar ground, namely the health team, and then move to the health of the population. Part I is somewhat theoretical and Part III may be new ground.

Individual health workers may be aware of certain concrete problems that hamper their effectiveness and may wish to solve them on their own, as far as possible.

For instance:

> You may find that a pain-reliever that you wish to dispense is out of stock. Presumably the need is to replenish stocks in time. Chapter 2 of Part III covers "Managing drugs" and the related exercises should help you in dealing with the problem.

> If in studying the chapter you find that the problem is a different one, e.g. lack of administrative authority to purchase drugs, you will also need to study this aspect before raising the matter with your supervisor.

A health worker in charge of the health care activities of a health team becomes aware of some fault in work organization that affects the team's efficiency.

For instance:

> For some weeks you have been behind schedule in the nutritional surveillance programme. Your team may come to the conclusion that its targets were unrealistic to begin with. Objectives and perhaps activities have to be replanned. After studying Chapter 1 (Planning health activities) of Part IV, the team decides on a series of working sessions to revise the plan for the next financial year. While revising the plan you realize that there may have been

something wrong in the way the budget for the nutrition programme was shown. Your next training workshop will deal with this matter.

A health worker who solves management problems easily as they arise wonders what other people find so difficult. In this case it may be advisable to begin by reading Part I and doing the corresponding exercises, and then to go on to items of specific interest.

Lay-out of the guide

This guide is divided into parts (I to IV) and each part (except Part I) into several chapters. Each chapter begins with a statement of learning objectives, which is a list of what the trainees should be able to do as a result of having studied the texts and done the exercises.

Each part contains a number of exercises after the last chapter. Possible solutions to these exercises are given at the end of the book, immediately before the Glossary.

Practise as you learn

Little can be gained by merely reading this book. It would be like reading a book on swimming in the middle of a desert. Only by applying in practice what is read can the skills of management be acquired.

Managing well makes work easier. It improves relations with colleagues and the service given to others; it makes life pleasanter and more rewarding and improves the quality of work. Managing well also leads to harmonious work; it lessens the irritations and frustrations that arise from confusion and poor organization.

> **TRY THE FOLLOWING EXERCISE**

Preliminary exercise: Diagnosing management problems

The statements on pages 7 and 8 describe some of the problems that may trouble a health worker. Read each statement and ask yourself whether you agree with it. Using the scale on the right side of the page, record the extent of your agreement with a tick (✓) — one for each statement. Allow 15 minutes to complete the exercise.

	I totally disagree	I tend to disagree	I don't know	I tend to agree	I fully agree
1) I know exactly what tasks I am expected to do at all times					
2) We report to the administration the things they like to hear.					
3) I regularly attend the scheduled staff meetings to review problems of implementation					
4) I have occasionally been behind schedule in delivering my services					
5) During field visits, our team leader always takes time to listen to our difficulties					
6) I have experienced shortages of government funds during the past year					
7) The targets we agreed upon with the community leaders are easily met					
8) Members of my team are fully cooperative					
9) My salary is regularly paid on time					
10) The communities I serve have expressed full appreciation of the services they received last year					
11) The statistics on the chart at the health centre are not up to date					

12) I am adequately
    trained for what I am
    doing

13) Some of my colleagues
    are not adequately
    trained for what we are
    doing

14) There are frequent
    arguments among
    members of the team
    about our different
    duties and
    responsibilities

15) Occasionally I cannot
    do my work because
    of shortage of
    supplies

16) Coordination with
    other government
    departments is quite
    easy

17) Our leader is not fully
    informed of what we
    do

18) My job description has
    been reviewed and
    updated in the last
    three years

19) My partners in the
    team are not always
    sure what my job is

20) I spend far too much
    time on recording and
    reporting

21) Our norms of perform-
    ance are quite realistic

22) Our objectives are
    never reached on time

How to interpret your answers

(*a*) Record here your "total disagreement" answers to statements
    1 3 5 7 8 9 10 12 16 18 21   (circle as applicable).

(*b*) Record here your "total agreement" answers to statements
    2 4 6 11 13 14 15 17 19 20 22   (circle as applicable).

(*c*) Record here your "I don't know" answers to statements (write numbers)

The circled entries under (*a*) and (*b*), and the numbers entered under (*c*), are likely problem areas that management could help solve or at least improve.

If you have circled 1, 4, 7, 21, 22, you probably need help in *planning*.

If you have circled 6, 8, 9, 12, 13, 14, 18, you probably need help in *organization*.

If you have circled 3, 16, 19, but also 1, 4, or 14, you probably need help in *direction*.

If you have circled 3, 5, 12, 13, you probably need help in *supervision*.

If the circled items were 6, 11, 15, 17, 20, you probably need help in the areas of *resources*, *monitoring* and *control*.

Items 2, 7 and 10 relate to *evaluation*.

If you have circled entries everywhere, then your trouble is the whole *management* field.

**GO ON TO THE TOPIC
YOU HAVE CHOSEN TO STUDY**

PART I

What is management?

CHAPTER 1

Concepts, definitions, principles and main functions of management

Management has been applied since the beginning of civilization and community living; it is not an invention of the 20th century. Whenever people have worked together in groups — to grow crops, to buy and sell, to wage war, to build a temple — there has been management.

Although management is so old and universal, it has no agreed definition; there are many definitions to choose from and readers can select their own to suit their purposes. Perhaps the shortest is:

Management is: getting things done

The principle underlying this definition is 'commitment to achievement', i.e. commitment to purposeful action, not to action for its own sake. To stress this notion of purpose the definition may be rewritten as follows: 'management is saying what one wants to be done, and then getting it done'. In other words, management ensures first that objectives are specified (i.e. states specifically what is to be achieved) and then that they are achieved.

Management by objectives

Deciding and saying what is to be accomplished is setting an objective (a goal, a purpose, an end, a target). There are many kinds of objective.

For instance:

> As leader of a health team, you may have set your objectives as follows.

> *Next year* in the village of Venka:

> — there will be no cases of diphtheria,
> — there will be one protected well for every ten families,
> — 60% of the pregnant women will attend prenatal clinics and be delivered by a midwife,
> — all known cases of tuberculosis will complete ten months' treatment with isoniazid.

> And *for the week ending 27 July* your team objectives at the Venka Health Centre might be:

> — to hold daily clinics from 9.00 a.m. to 3.00 p.m.
> — to complete the drugs inventory and order a new supply from the district health officer,
> — to hold a staff discussion on child malnutrition in Venka,
> — to have the jeep serviced at 45 000 km.

Some of these objectives refer to aspects of a population's health at some later time, some refer to services that will be made available to the population, others refer to the coverage of some eligible group, still others refer to tasks that will be performed during a particular period. However, all should state:

— what is to be done
— how much is to be done
— where it is to be done
— when it is to be completed
— the standard by which it will be possible to tell whether, or the extent to which, it has been achieved.

(The reader may take time to check whether these are true of the above example.)

Why should such objectives be set? An educationalist once gave a humorous answer to this question but it contains a deep truth: "If you're not sure where you're going, you're liable to end up someplace else."[1]

Of course, merely saying where you intend to go does not take you there; nor is saying that you intend to produce some result enough for the result to happen. However, it helps, in several different ways. It helps in deciding the methods you will use to produce the result. It helps those who are to produce the result to organize, distribute and coordinate their efforts. It helps in determining when the intended result is being achieved or has been achieved. In other words, a clear statement of objectives is essential for effectiveness.

Effectiveness is the degree to which an objective is being, or has been, achieved; it is something that management tries to improve.

For instance:

> If a health team sets itself the objective of 100 children to be immunized against diphtheria during the following week, and succeeds in immunizing 95, the work has been managed effectively. (However, if an epidemic of diphtheria were to occur a few weeks later, how would you judge the team's performance?)
>
> If, by the end of 1995, the population of Venka has one protected well for every 22 families, and the objective was one for every 10 families, it seems very likely that those in charge did not manage their programme effectively.
>
> If the health centre at Venka remains closed for two days during the week ending 27 July, can it be said that the objective of holding daily clinics has been achieved effectively?

TRY EXERCISE 1 ON PAGE 32

The management principle that underlies the comparison of objectives with their achievement in order to judge effectiveness is known as 'learning from experience'. It derives from and justifies — proves the value of — the first management principle, namely, management by objectives.

---

[1] Mager, R. F. *Preparing instructional objectives,* 2nd ed. Belmont, CA, Pitman Learning Inc., 1975.

Learning from experience

How is this principle applied? When there is a gap between objectives and results (or achievement), management analyses why only the observed results were achieved, and why they fell short of the set objectives. Some causes can be easily remedied, and action is taken accordingly. Others cannot be removed in the short term and are then called constraints. Management learns from this process and uses what it has learned in its further decisions for achieving its objectives. This process is sometimes called 'feedback' (of information from experience to decision for action). Other kinds of feedback that allow management to learn from experience are discussed in Part IV, Chapter 3.

A second reason for specifying objectives clearly is that it enables management and health workers to decide *how* to achieve them. In other words, stating the objective, or *end*, helps in selecting the *means* of achieving it.

Sometimes, however, it is not clear which are ends and which are means.

When a pump has been installed, when a traditional birth attendant has been retrained, when a guide for primary-health-care management has been produced, are these ends or means?

When people have accepted the use of latrines, when children have been immunized, when health workers evaluate their own effectiveness, can we talk of ends or of means?

The answer is, of course, both. Every end may be seen as a means to a higher end, almost indefinitely: trained staff are a means of delivering better services; better services, in turn, are a means of improving a community's health; better health is a means of ensuring better quality of life. The following definition of management mentions both ends and means:

Management is: **getting things done through people**

This does not mean that someone (a manager) orders and others (people) do what they are ordered to do, although this is often what happens. It means, rather, that people are the most important means, or resource, for getting things done. Consequently Part II of this guide — Working with people, or the health-team approach — deals with people (or human resources).

TRY EXERCISE 2 ON PAGE 33

Getting things done through people means that people must work, performing certain activities and tasks to reach certain ends or objectives. When we are concerned with how *means* are used to reach *ends*, we are concerned with efficiency.

Efficiency is about reaching ends by only the necessary means or by the least wasteful use of means. It is a measure of the relation between the results obtained and the effort expended (by the health team, for example). This concept has many implications for the use of resources, as will be seen later; here the focus is on people, or human resources, and on the way they work.

Almost any work involves more than one person. As soon as two or more people are involved in work or activity, two complementary principles must be applied by management, namely *division of labour* and *convergence of work*.

Division of labour

When work is divided, or distributed, among members of a group, and the work is directed and coordinated, the group becomes a team. In a team, and generally when there is specialization and division of labour, with each category of staff exercising its own skills towards achieving the objectives, management consists in assigning a balanced proportion of each kind of staff to the work to be done.

Efficiency implies that all necessary means (but no more than necessary) are used to achieve objectives and that, if there is a choice of equally effective means, the least expensive is chosen.

The team approach is the way in which management attempts to bring about balance among the different members of the team and the work they do.

For instance:

> For a surgeon to perform an operation someone must give the anaesthetic, someone must lay out the instruments, someone must ensure that the instruments and the theatre clothes have been sterilized, electricians must assure the power supply, and various other kinds of staff must be responsible for other tasks.

The general principle of management illustrated by this example is the principle of division of labour: work must be shared by, or divided among, a number of different categories of technically skilled people.

As pointed out on page 15, one of the advantages of defining objectives and considering resources is that this helps in deciding *how* to reach the objectives, i.e. the *activities* needed to achieve them and the methods and organization that will enable people to work harmoniously towards the objectives, while using resources efficiently. The study of work activities and the organization of work relations form a major area of management. Its governing principle is that of *convergence of work*.

Convergence of work

Convergence of work means that the activities of the various people who do the work come together in the achievement of objectives. The activities should be designed, assigned and directed in such a way that they support each other in moving towards a common goal. It also implies that working relations — the ways in which the members of a team interact with one another — should contribute to the success of each activity, and thus to general effectiveness.

In general, health activities are studied, described and performed under three main headings, namely:

— service activities
— development activities
— support activities.

A service activity (e.g. immunization) usually requires some preceding development activity (e.g. training of immunizers), and some continuous support activity (e.g. provision of supplies). These three kinds of activity need to be managed so as to bring about convergence of work, balance of resources and harmonious work relations, and ultimately the intended results.

Specific work activities must be brought into logical relations with one another.

For instance:

> To provide services, trained staff are needed. To train staff, certain objectives are set. To achieve these objectives, various preliminary

development activities are carried out, also in relation to one another, e.g. designing a curriculum, preparing learning materials, selecting trainees, recruiting trainers.

Activities must also have a time (or temporal) relation or sequence.

For instance:

> Trainers can be recruited first, and asked to prepare the curriculum and the learning materials, and then to select trainees and begin teaching. However, other time sequences are possible. (Can you suggest one?)

> Also, training can begin either before staff recruitment (and therefore before beginning to provide the services), or after staff recruitment, when training is given 'on-the-job', i.e. at the same time as services are provided.

Frequency is an aspect of the time relationship. In the work of a health team, some activities (such as certain development activities) occur only once or rarely, some (such as services) occur more often, and some (such as support) occur continually.

There is also a place (or spatial) relation between activities.

For instance:

> Services are given in the homes of families (e.g. treatment of illness); on-the-job training may take place elsewhere in the district; formal training is given in a classroom at the health centre, or at a training college; the curriculum may be designed in the capital city; etc.

TRY EXERCISE 3 ON PAGE 34

Another useful definition is:

Management is: **the efficient use of resources**

It is well recognized in health work, as in other kinds of activity, that the different types of resources used for achieving objectives must be carefully balanced. Use of the team approach to bring about balance among the different people (human resources) concerned has already been mentioned. However, other resources must also be managed to achieve objectives; examples are materials (equipment and supplies) and money (without which people and materials often would not be available). Beyond these 'three Ms' — manpower, materials, money — there are time and information, which the health team must also have. These other types of resource must also be kept in balance.

For instance:

> If there is insufficient equipment (e.g. syringes) or a shortage of supplies (e.g. petrol), a health team may not be able to reach its immunization target.

> When money runs short, salaries cannot be paid on time and staff morale drops, and this may result in targets not being reached.

A prime concern of management is therefore to ensure adequate funds and stocks of materials to permit the staff to provide the planned services. This is one meaning of "efficient use of resources" in the above definition of management.

If all resources were plentiful and free, the concept of efficiency might have no practical importance. However, some — often many — resources are scarce and costly.

For instance:

> Jaya Province has an ample supply of trained people to staff the health services. But the local authorities are poor and their budget does not allow them to fill vacancies without cutting down on supplies, such as petrol for transport or essential drugs (both of which are imported, and therefore costly).

This is a typically difficult position for management, which illustrates one more concept — economy — and one more principle — substitution of resources.

In everyday life some commodities become scarce, either because production or supply falls or because demand for them rises. As a result, they become more expensive. When a commodity becomes scarce or more expensive, ordinary people buy less of it; in other words, they economize. The concept of *economy* — or careful use of resources — is applied by almost everyone in daily life, with more or less success. The related principle, *substitution of resources*, is also widely applied.

Often, when the resources normally used to provide services become scarce or too expensive, different resources or a different balance of resources may be used to produce the intended results.

For instance:

> When purchasing food for a hospital kitchen, cheap produce in season can be substituted for other similar but more expensive food if it is equally nourishing.

> When petrol continues to go up in price, bicycles may be substituted, at least partly, for motorized transport. The savings on petrol, vehicle maintenance and drivers may be better spent on more field staff (perhaps saving time previously lost on travel), thus achieving the same coverage of the population as before.

This leads to the fifth principle of management, *substitution of resources.*

Substitution of resources

One particular type of substitution of resources is labour substitution (e.g. using trained auxiliary personnel or volunteers for tasks formerly undertaken by professionals). This subject is discussed in Part IV, Step 5. A familiar example of resource distribution in health management is the use of generic drugs (in countries where generic drugs are reliable) instead of brand-name preparations, which are usually much more expensive.

TRY EXERCISE 4 ON PAGE 36

One more definition may be considered briefly, which brings together many of the points discussed so far:

Management is: **getting people to work harmoniously together and to make efficient use of resources to achieve objectives.**

This definition stresses the need to ensure that people work well and cooperatively together. Working relations are a major concern of managers

The working relations between people are usually described as *functional* and *structural. Functional relations* derive directly from the technical nature of the work, and where, when, and in what sequence it is done. An example is the working relationship between the members of a surgical team. *Structural relations* pertain to administrative rules and standards, and in particular to the authority and responsibility assigned to individuals — for example, who engages and dismisses staff, how much a medical officer may spend without referring to higher authorities, or to whom the public health nurse must submit her reports and accounts.

The two key concepts that underlie functional and structural relations within a health team are *responsibility* and *authority*, which can hardly be considered separately in the day-to-day management of team-work.

For instance:

> A member of the staff of a health centre who is made responsible for the immunization coverage of the district must be authorized: to requisition vaccines from the central cold-storage depot; to order transport from the vehicle pool for the immunization team; to have the refrigerator repaired if necessary; to replace leaky syringes and used needles with new materials from the stores; etc. Otherwise, the immunization programme will not be carried out properly.

or:

> An officer who is responsible for "directing and supervising" staff, but who has no say in matters of their leave, transfer or promotion, would not be able to fulfil his or her responsibilities.

The management principle that derives directly from the need to associate responsibility and authority may be stated as *functions determine structure*.

Functions determine structure

When work is clearly defined, i.e. the *function* and duties of individual members of the team are clearly defined and known to all, the working relations (the *structure*) follow.

TRY EXERCISE 5 ON PAGE 37

However, what is the exact nature of *authority*? One more definition of management will help clarify this point:

Management is: **to make decisions**

This definition is more general than those given earlier. It stresses the most important element of management, namely *decision-making*. A decision is a choice between two or more courses of action. It can be a resolve to act — "this shall be done" — or, sometimes, not to act — "this shall go on as before". Some decisions deal with quantity — "more of this, less of that, none of the other"; some deal with quality — "higher coverage, better services". In management terms a decision is an answer to a question about possible courses of action, an answer that can be stated simply as: yes, no, more, none. "I don't know" in this context is *indecision*.

The authority of a member of the health team, then, may be defined simply as the decisions which that member may make. A common failing of management is that no one is clearly responsible for some urgently needed decision, or that someone is responsible but has not been given the necessary authority to act.

For instance:

> The team's jeep has broken down in the bush. The driver, after securing police watch over the vehicle, reports to his officer-in-charge, who is "responsible for the maintenance and upkeep of transport". But the breakdown truck belongs to the Ministry of Transport and Public Works, and the charge for picking up the jeep is likely to be more than $200. The officer-in-charge has authority to spend up to $10 on repairs, and the district health officer up to $100 only. The provincial health administration has already spent its budget allotment for transport. The questions are: *who* is the decision-maker, and *where* is he or she?

A major concern in working relations is to enable decisions to be made, where and when necessary, by the most suitable person. Any member of a health team may be called upon to make a decision at one time or another, especially when the team leader is absent, or otherwise the team would be paralysed.

It can happen that a health worker who follows the rules strictly does nothing, and is then blamed for doing nothing, say in an emergency. What is needed then is the application of the principle of *delegation*.

Delegation

Delegation takes place when someone with authority 'lends' the authority to another person, conditionally or not, so as to enable that person to take responsibility when the need arises. This management principle has been stated with a humorous twist in the words: "Never do yourself what another can do for you as well as you would". This advice is for the busy manager, but it could well apply in anybody's family life, as well as in the performance of the tasks of any member of a health team.

To decide between different courses of action *information* and *decision rules* are needed.

For instance:

> A management *decision* for health team X is whether to transfer the responsibility for intravenous injections from one staff category (A) to another (B). The relevant decision *rule* might be: "If intravenous injections take more than 20% of A's work time, and if B, after training, can give ten consecutive intravenous injections without fault, then A may authorize B to take over this task". *Information* is needed to show that the injections take over 20% of A's time, that B has been trained, and that B has passed the test.

Another element of decision-making is ensuring that the decision, once taken, is made known to all concerned. This is *communication*. Many people would even say that all concerned should know beforehand that a decision is about to be made. Often, knowledge about the need for a decision, and taking part in making it, are the best assurances that the decision will subsequently be acted upon. One thing is essential, however, and that is communication between those who make decisions, those who implement them, and the people affected by the decisions. At least, the decision itself should be communicated, but normally the supporting information, the decision rules, and how the decision is to be implemented, should also be included.

TRY EXERCISE 6 ON PAGE 39

Of course, management need not know everything that takes place. In particular, a programme that runs well does not usually call for control decisions. What is essential is to be informed about exceptions, i.e. things that do not go well and may require urgent decisions. The management principle that deals with information is *management by exception*.

Management by exception

Management by exception means two things:

First: *be selective.* Do not become overloaded with routine and unnecessary information. Keep your mind available for critical information, on which you will be required to *act.*

For instance:

> If you were in charge of fifty beds, you would not want to know every day every patient's blood pressure, temperature, pulse rate, respiration rate, bowel movements, volume of fluids passed, etc. Just one of these elements of information might be all you would need to watch in each case to manage most patients effectively and efficiently.

Second: *make big decisions first.* To be overloaded with petty decisions may result in more important ones being neglected, or what has been called "postponing decisions until they become unnecessary". In short, management by exception means selectivity in information and priority in decision.

Shortest decision-path

The last management principle discussed in this chapter, the principle of the shortest decision-path, deals with the issue: *who* should make *which* decision? (and often *when* and *where*, as well). Answering this type of question will help in clarifying the question of *delegation* of authority referred to earlier.

Applying this principle means that decisions are made as close as possible in time and place to the object of the decision and to those affected by it. This saves time and work (e.g. in transmitting information) and also ensures that decisions can take full account of the circumstances which make the decisions necessary and in which they are put into effect.

The main functions of management

A function may be defined as: **a group of activities with a common purpose.**

Management consists of many functions thus defined. A health team has three main management functions: *planning, implementation* and *evaluation.*

One way of determining what constitutes management functions is to review the principles set out earlier in this chapter and note the various functions that they imply.

Thus, the principle of *management by objectives* requires the specification of *what* and *how much* is to be done, and *where* and *when* it is to be done. Each of these four questions needs one or more planning decisions. The sum of the planning decisions constitutes the *planning* function of management in a health team.

The principle of *delegation* is concerned with authority and responsibility, i.e. with functional relations between people working together to achieve some purpose. The types of decision involved are concerned with the organization of working relations so as to ensure effective and efficient work, i.e. implementation. Organization decisions are part of the *implementation* function of management.

Applying the principle of *learning from experience* requires the analysis of gaps between desired results and actual results, or achievement, and the use in decision-making of the information obtained from the analysis. This is, in other words, a measurement and a judgement of performance, or the *evaluation* function of management, a function that contributes greatly to the success of a health team.

As an aid to memory these three broad functions of management are sometimes presented graphically as follows:

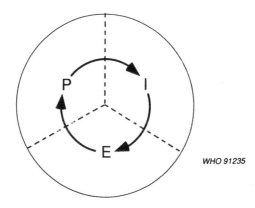

WHO 91235

The diagram shows *planning* (P), *implementation* (I) and *evaluation* (E) as three parts of a 'pie'. What matters, however, are the arrows, which link the three functions to emphasize the continuous cycle of management.

These three functions of management, as applied to primary health care, are described in detail, in terms of their specific activities, in Part IV of this guide:

— planning in Chapter 1, page 267
— implementation in Chapter 2, page 316
— evaluation in Chapter 3, page 341

TRY EXERCISE 7 ON PAGE 40

Highlights of Part I

For *effectiveness*
Management states objectives and learns from experience.

For *efficiency*
Management distributes work in such a way that the activities of the different members of the health team converge (come together).

For *economy*
Management finds and obtains the resources needed to achieve its objectives, or makes the best use of the resources that are available if it cannot obtain the most suitable at reasonable cost. When resources become scarce or too expensive it substitutes less expensive resources.

For *harmonious functional and structural relations*
Management assigns and delegates responsibility and authority.

Management is decision-making based on adequate information, sound rules and good communication.

Management has three main functions: planning, implementation, and evaluation.

All staff share management tasks.

Exercises

Exercises — general information

Each exercise has a number, followed in parenthesis by the designation of the Part (in Roman numerals) and the Chapter (in Arabic numerals) to which it refers.

The objective of each exercise is stated at the beginning of the exercise.

The exercises can be done before studying the corresponding chapters (to find out whether study is needed), during study (to reinforce what has been learned), or after study (to assess whether something new has been learned).

It is recommended that the exercises are done first individually and then in a group. Most of the exercises indicate these two steps and are so designed that group work by the health team cannot fruitfully take place without individual preparation by each health worker. If group work is placed on the agenda of a staff meeting, the staff members involved should be given time to prepare themselves. Individual preparation for an exercise may require 35–40 minutes and group discussion 45–90 minutes.

The exercises are not of uniform difficulty or complexity. Teachers and supervisors may use or recommend them selectively for health workers at varying levels of education and experience, and at different times and even for different purposes (e.g. to determine training needs). Individual health workers may use them in the same way and for similar purposes.

Illustrations of possible solutions to some of the exercises are given at the end of the book. For certain of the exercises, however, the 'solutions' are in their performance, whether they are meant for individual or group work.

Exercises for Part I

Exercise 1 (I.1) Management by objectives

Objective: To be able to explain why it is necessary to define objectives, and to state ten important objectives of the health team.

Individual work

Write down what you think your health team's objectives are in the field of primary health care:

—

—

—

—

—

Mark with a cross (×) those objectives that the team is currently pursuing.

Prepare yourself to show how such objectives help in the management of the team's work, and note down a few key words you would use in a group discussion of this topic:

—

—

—

—

Group work

Compare the lists of objectives prepared by the individual health workers and record the ten current objectives most often mentioned. Through discussion of these ten objectives decide which of them pertain to the following categories:

— the health of the community
— the services (to be) delivered
— the tasks that health workers must perform
— the resources used.

Discuss the relation between objectives in the different categories, what should be done about 'objectives' that do not fit into any of the categories, whether some objectives are missing, and what should be done about objectives that are not being pursued.

Then review the health workers' ideas on how stating objectives helps in the management of the work, discuss these ideas, and record all points of agreement.

Exercise 2 (I.1) Learning from experience

Objective: To be able to share with other members of the team your experiences in the achievement of objectives.

Individual work

Try to remember something useful and important that you have learned from experience in primary health care. Answer the questions:

What new knowledge have you gained? . . . .

What new attitude have you developed? . . . .

What new skill have you acquired? . . . .

For what activity or task were those useful? . . . .

To what objective were they related? . . . .

What proof have you that learning was useful? . . . .

. . . .

With whom did you share the experience? . . . .

How did the sharing take place? . . . .

Who else applies what they learned from this shared experience? . . . .

Prepare yourself to contribute to a group discussion on how the team could best ensure the sharing of experience as part of its continuing education.

Group work

Review individual health workers' accounts of learning from experience. First, write down the objectives to which the learning related, and discover from discussion which of them are missing. Second, determine what are the activities or tasks for which learning was found useful, and write them down in relation to the objectives to which they refer. Third, write down, next to the relevant objectives and activities, the tests that will be used to assess the usefulness of the learning.

Then review the content of the learning from experience:

What concepts were learned or better understood?
What experiences led to changed attitudes, and what changes took place in attitudes?
What new skills were acquired or existing skills improved?

The discussion of these points should highlight the relation between competence and performance.

Then consider the process of sharing experience. List those who took part, and those who apply the learning; then list the circumstances and methods of sharing experience.

Finally, review suggestions from the health workers for improvements to the current means of learning from experience, so as to increase the sharing and use of experience, and ultimately the effectiveness of primary health care.

Exercise 3 (I.1) Task analysis in team-work

Objective: To be able to analyse tasks and assignments in the team, and to show how team-work can improve efficiency.

Individual work

Think of a particular primary health care activity you do well, and list the tasks involved. (*Hint*: think what you have to do first, second, etc. through to the last task.)

Then think of any other person associated with that activity. (*Hint*: do you need support, communication, etc.?)

Record the task in the left-hand column of the table below, and the people who help in doing the work in the top row of the table. Then try to show with a tick (✓) in the appropriate places *who* takes part in doing *which* tasks.

Finally, prepare yourself to contribute to a group discussion on how task analysis and assignment can contribute to improving the team's efficiency.

Activity.						
Tasks ╲ Name and designation	Myself	Other people helping with the work				
		1)	2)	3)	4)	
a)						
b)						
c)						
d)						
e)						
f)						
g)						
h)						
i)						
j)						

Group work

First review the activities analysed by individual health workers, and select one with which to start the discussion. Then discuss the listed tasks one by one, and if necessary add, delete, remove or modify terms used to describe the tasks; put them in logical order. Discuss the list of people helping with the work, clarifying and completing it if necessary. Review the task assignment proposed, discuss it and, if there is agreement on necessary changes, modify it.

Repeat the same review and discussion for the other activities (analysed by the other health workers). Compare the assignments proposed by different workers to see whether they match, and make necessary adjustments. Discuss how such analysis can help increase the services the team provides and improve their quality by making the best use of the staff. Try to answer the question: what other analyses need to be done to complete the discussions on efficiency?

Exercise 4 (I.1) Using resources efficiently

Objective: To be able to analyse the use of resources in primary health care, and show how a balanced use of resources can improve efficiency.

Individual work

List the resources that the team has used in its primary health care activities:

—

—

—

—

—

Then think of a primary health care activity you perform regularly. (*Hint*: it may be the same as in Exercise 3.) Check which resources you used in each task: record these in the table below.

Recall instances of shortage of one resource necessary for a particular task. Think of the consequences of the shortage, and write a few words about the experience:

Resource: . . . .   Needed for task: . . . .

How did this shortage affect other resources?. . . . .

. . . .

How did it affect other tasks? . . . .

. . . .

How did it affect the activity? . . . .

. . . .

How did it affect the achievement of objectives? . . . .

. . . .

How did it affect the cost of services? . . . .

. . . .

Prepare yourself to take part in a group discussion on this topic, especially to suggest ways of remedying such shortages of resources.

Tasks	Resources used in performing these tasks				
	1)	2)	3)	4)	5)
a) b) c) d) e) f)					

Group work

Review the resources listed by the health workers and summarize them in four to six groups. Review the use of various resources for different tasks and compare the costs involved. Then select one of the instances of resource shortage; listen to and discuss the health worker's conclusions about the effects of the shortage on other resources, and on tasks, activities, etc. Consider alternative remedial actions, either for resolving the shortage or for adjusting other resources, or the task, the activity or the objective itself. Review other instances of resource shortage in a similar way. In each case try to estimate the effect of the shortage in terms of the achievement of the objective and of wastage of human resources, as a basis for remedial action.

Exercise 5 (I.1) Assigning management tasks

Objective: To be able to describe the distribution of responsibility for management functions in the health team, and show how it affects the structural relations of the members of the team.

Individual work

Review the previous exercises to find instances of management tasks. (*Hint*: review the learning objectives, the steps in the exercises, and the tables produced.) List a few management tasks in the table below. (The last task — "Supervision of above"— is an example of a management task not mentioned in the previous exercises: it has been added here to make this exercise more interesting and useful.) List the members of the team by name and designation, and show — by a cross (×) in the appropriate box — *who* is responsible for *which* management task. (If persons outside the team are involved, record them under: "People outside the team".)

Select a few management tasks you have assigned yourself. Think of any difficulties you have had in performing these tasks, and write them down:

. . . .
. . . .
. . . .
. . . .
. . . .

Prepare yourself to discuss how to overcome these difficulties in your management work.

Management tasks	Who is responsible within the health team?					People outside the team
	1)	2)	3)	4)	5)	
a) b) c) d) e) f) Supervision of above						

Group work

Review the management tasks suggested by individual health workers and combine them in a list as duties of the entire team. Discuss the assignment by the different health workers of management responsibilities for themselves, and record them. Then, taking each team member in turn, discuss responsibilities as assigned by the other team members, and record those on which there is general agreement. Note unclear assignments, for referral to senior staff.

Then review the difficulties that the health workers have in doing their work. Was the assignment not clear, not adequately described, not communicated, or not accepted? Was the task not included in a work-plan, not performed for lack of some resource, performed but without result, etc.? Note the frequency of such difficulties.

Then discuss individual suggestions for improving structural relations with a view to improving management. Note any measures agreed upon, for submission to senior staff.

Exercise 6 (I.1) Rules for decision-making

Objective: To be able to name the decisions you are called upon to make in your work, to recall the decision rules involved, and to find the information you need in order to make them.

Individual work

Try to remember some decisions you have to make in the course of your work, and note them down.

—
—
—
—
—

Check the following list to see whether you have remembered all the kinds of decision you make: use of space, procedures to be followed, use of time, assignment of tasks, use of equipment, priorities among objectives, use of supplies, working conditions.

If necessary, complete your list of decisions, then recall an instance where you could *not* make a necessary decision.

The decision was: . . . .

It concerned activity: . . . .

Try to identify why you did not make the decision:

Were you:

— responsible for it?   Yes/No/Don't know
— authorized to make it?   Yes/No/Don't know

Did you:

— know the rule to be applied?   Yes/No
— have norms to refer to?   Yes/No
— have the information you needed?   Yes/No

The consequence of not making the decision was: . . . .
. . . .

If you never make decisions, why not?   . . . .
. . . .

Group work

Review and discuss the nature of decisions made by all individual staff and by each staff category. Note the frequency of each type of decision and record the complete list. Then review and discuss, one by one, the instances of decisions *not* made, beginning with the circumstances and the consequences, continuing with the reasons given by the health workers, and concluding in each case with the reasons as seen by the team as a whole.

Agree for each of the cases studied:

— to whom the issue should be referred—*responsibility*
— how the issue should be presented—*information needed*
— alternative suggestions — *decision rules.*

Exercise 7 (I.1) Relating resources, activities and results

Objective: To be able to explain how resources, activities and results are interrelated.

Individual or group work

Study the diagram on page 41. Make a large copy and fill in the headings you think describe best the activities of a (your) health team. List the main resources the team uses in carrying out the activities, and name some of the results it achieves (or should achieve).

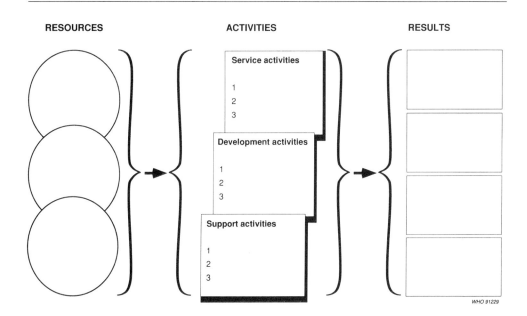

RESOURCES   ACTIVITIES   RESULTS

Service activities

1
2
3

Development activities

1
2
3

Support activities

1
2
3

WHO 91229

NOW FILL IN
THE EVALUATION SHEET
THAT FOLLOWS

Evaluation of Part I

On the 0 to 5 scale, mark with a tick (✓) the extent of your agreement with the following statements:

Reading material is:

relevant to my work	0--/--/--/--/--/--5
useful for my work	0--/--/--/--/--/--5
difficult to understand	0--/--/--/--/--/--5
too time-consuming	0--/--/--/--/--/--5

Individual exercises are:

relevant to the subject	0--/--/--/--/--/--5
useful as means of learning	0--/--/--/--/--/--5
difficult to perform	0--/--/--/--/--/--5
too time-consuming	0--/--/--/--/--/--5

Group exercises are:

relevant to the team's work	0--/--/--/--/--/--5
useful for the team's work	0--/--/--/--/--/--5
difficult to perform	0--/--/--/--/--/--5
too time-consuming	0--/--/--/--/--/--5

I have acquired:

new knowledge	0--/--/--/--/--/--5
new attitudes	0--/--/--/--/--/--5
new skills	0--/--/--/--/--/--5

PART II

Working with people, or the health-team approach

"People are the most important resource of any country. . ." (*Primary Health Care. Report of the International Conference on Primary Health Care, Alma-Ata, USSR, 6–12 September 1978.* Geneva, World Health Organization, 1978.)

Introduction

People may be cooks, teachers, engineers, nurses or medical assistants, but at some time during the course of their work they will also be *managers*.

The quality of what is produced — a tasty meal, an interesting lesson, a safe machine, or a successful health programme — depends on a person or group of people. In other words, *only people make things happen*. There may be money, equipment, materials and techniques, but none of these can perform a task, either simple or complex, without a person or group of people to initiate action.

A health worker with management responsibilities deals with people and things. Both are important, but since 80% of health budgets is spent on salaries and staff benefits, and people matter more than things, effective supervisors will give much more attention to the people with whom they work than to the things they handle.

Managing people is more complex than managing things. Things cannot think or answer back; above all, they cannot feel, they are insensitive. But to work harmoniously with people demands understanding and skill. People like to feel useful and appreciated and may become discouraged when they are ignored or unjustly criticized. When people are helped and their work problems are understood, the quality of their work improves.

Efficient ways of working and regular pay are not enough to keep people satisfied at work. The work must also be interesting and stimulating; working conditions, the environment, relations among team members and between the community and the health team are major factors in determining work satisfaction. The person in charge of a health team has an important responsibility to be sympathetic and helpful to the other health workers and to try to maintain a relaxed and happy working atmosphere.

The following chapters discuss different aspects of working with people as a colleague, as a leader or as a member of the community. Better health care depends largely on efficient management, i.e. making the best use of available resources. But management depends on people, and good management can help a team to work together harmoniously and efficiently. Five ways of achieving this are described in the chapters that follow:

— by setting and sharing objectives (Chapter 2, Section 2.1);
— by encouraging good personal relations (Chapter 2, Sections 2.4 and 4.4);

— by distributing tasks (Chapter 3);
— by coordinating the activities of the team (Chapter 3, Section 3.2); and
— by applying sound organization principles (Chapter 3, Section 3.2).

CHAPTER 1

The health team and its work in the community

Learning objectives

After studying this chapter and doing Exercises 8–13 on pages 117–123, the health worker should be able to:

— define "health team"

— create a work team, using principles of interpersonal relations

— establish relations with the community.

The health team has been defined as a group of people who share a common health goal and common objectives, determined by community needs, to the achievement of which each member of the team contributes, in accordance with his or her competence and skill and in coordination with the functions of others.[1] The manner and degree of such cooperation will vary and has to be determined by each society according to its own needs and resources. There can be no universally applicable composition of a health team.

The members of a health team include *all* those working together; for example, the supporting staff — clerks, drivers, cleaners — are all part of the team. It is important that their work and contributions be recognized as well as those of the technical staff (medical assistants, nurses and community health workers).

There are many different kinds of health team, depending on the type of health work that teams undertake. Some are specialist health teams, such

---

[1] *Glossary of terms used in the "Health for all" Series No. 1–8.* Geneva, World Health Organization, 1984 ("Health for all Series", No. 9), p. 13.

as mobile teams — that travel from place to place dealing with one disease (such as leprosy or tuberculosis) — or surgical teams in hospitals. In this guide the health team refers mainly to a group of health workers serving a population that may consist of many communities spread over a large area. The team works with the communities in providing essential health care.

A health team usually has a base: team members may work together in one building, such as a health centre, where equipment is kept and some clinics are held. From this base they visit communities to deal with health problems, undertake school health work, hold clinics, or follow up patients in their homes. Sometimes the team may have no such base but may operate as a mobile team in various communities, or individuals may work in separate villages but within the framework of an area programme. A health team may also include a village health worker chosen by the village people and based in the village.

The principles of interdependence and teamwork are the same in all cases but their applications will be different.

1.1 The health team, primary health care and community participation

The health team exists for the community. The community has health needs and it is the function of the health team to respond to those needs. No one person can acquire all the necessary skills, or have enough time, to do everything that must be done to satisfy the health needs of even a small community. Therefore, people have to work in teams to get the work done.

The aim of a community health team, working from a base (called a health centre or a clinic) must be to help communities attain and maintain health by means of essential or primary health care. Too often, the health team is concerned only with those in the community who come to the health centre or with those whom they meet in the field. However, community health care must also be concerned with the health problems of those people who do not or cannot come to the health centre and do not therefore benefit from the services available there.

Primary health care is essential health care made universally available to individuals and families. It includes those services that promote health such as keeping a clean environment, a good water supply, care of women during pregnancy and childbirth, nutrition of children, immunization, and early treatment of disease. Such services depend for their success on the active participation or involvement of the communities and individuals concerned. The health team has an essential role in such services but cannot alone ensure their success.

To achieve its aim a health team must be able to encourage, stimulate and support community participation, i.e. help people to rely as much as possible on their own efforts and resources to meet their health needs. One important way in which a community takes responsibility for its health is by appointing its own primary health care workers, and it then becomes a duty of the health team from the health centre to train and support these workers.

The members of the team should also work closely with workers from other sectors concerned with community welfare and development, such as teachers, agriculture extension workers, community development workers, and religious leaders.

To work well as a team, and to be able to stimulate and encourage community action and support village-level primary health care workers, the leader and other members of the health team need the skills of leadership and organization. These skills can be learned. People can learn to work well and together as a group, but the health team must use the skills of leadership and organization in cooperating with the community in its health and developmental activities. It is here that these skills are most usefully applied.

A health team must:

— understand and communicate with the community;
— encourage community participation in identifying problems and seeking solutions; and
— work in the community, i.e. in health centres, community meeting-places, work-places, schools and people's homes.

To establish relations with the community a health team does not tell the people what to do or give them orders; rather it works *with* people. To establish good relations with the community a health worker or health team follows four steps:

— listen, learn and understand;
— talk, discuss and decide;
— encourage, organize and participate; and
— inform.

Listen, learn and understand

Every community is different. Even in the same country, there are differences between local communities. To work with people and help them it is essential to understand their way of life.

There are many details to learn about the way people live, and they can be learned only by living among the people, listening and watching. It is not good to ask too many questions; this annoys people.

Health workers may observe and learn about communities under the following headings:

— work and living standards (community resources)
— family life
— social and political structure
— population structure
— values, beliefs and customs
— health attitudes.

Work and living standards

How do people get food? How do they earn money? Are they farm workers, fishermen, cattle-farmers, estate workers, factory workers? How do they spend their free time? Do they work at night?

Who works, the men or the women or both? Do children work? How many of the children attend school?

Is the community poor? Is it becoming less poor or more poor? Is its standard of living higher or lower than the average for the country? Are there good markets, good roads? Is there a clean water supply? Is there electricity, a telephone service, a bus service?

How do families live? What are the houses like? Do they have a system of sanitation? Are the houses infested?

Family life

What are the qualities of the relationships within the family? Who makes decisions? Is the family system an extended one? How many children are there in the average family? How are the children fed and how are they taught?

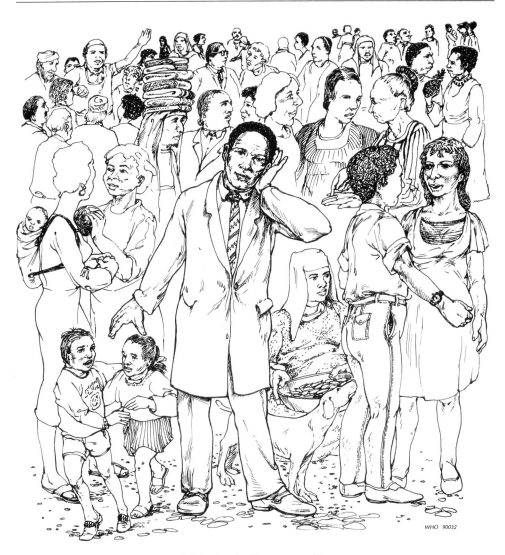

WHO 90032

Listening to the community

Social and political structure

Who are the community leaders? How do they become leaders? Who makes the decisions? Is the political structure authoritarian (power from above) or democratic (the people are consulted)? (See Chapter 2, Section 2.4, on styles of supervision.)

Do people meet in the market, at water-supply points, in clubs, at religious ceremonies, in their houses?

Population structure

Are there many old people? How many children are being born? Are there many women of childbearing age? Are there very few young adults because most have left the village to work in the towns?

Values, beliefs and customs

In every community there are sets of beliefs about life, which come from tradition and religion. There are customs that regulate how people behave towards one another, such as giving respect to elders, demanding obedience from children. Customs also determine behaviour in marriage and childbirth and at death.

Values show what people think are most important. For example, some people place very high value on clothes and personal appearance, some on dancing and social occasions, and others on polite forms and manners in social relations. Health workers need to understand very fully the beliefs, customs and values of the people.

Health attitudes

What are the common beliefs about the causes of sickness? What treatments are used within the family? Are there herbal remedies? Are there traditional healers? What traditional methods are used? Are there special beliefs about childbirth, breast-feeding and weaning? Are there food taboos during pregnancy? What is the attitude to child-spacing or family planning?

Talk, discuss and decide

The next step for the health worker is to lead the community towards recognizing its health problems and putting them in order of priority. Discussions can be both informal and formal. Informal discussions with families and people in the markets and shops will show what concerns people most. Informal discussions with political and religious leaders and with other government agencies will produce further ideas. After many informal talks it should be possible to make a list of the main problems that concern the community.

At this stage, a formal meeting convened by a community leader could be held to try to decide which are the most serious problems and what can be done about them. This could be difficult and several meetings might be needed before any clear decision can be reached. In this way the people are encouraged to participate in solving their own health problems. However, health staff should be cautious in such meetings, as community leaders are likely to try to persuade the people to agree with them about which problems should be given priority. Not everyone in a community has a say, and some important health problems may be forgotten, rejected or neglected by the leaders, particularly when they concern only certain people in the community, whose views might be seen as questioning the priorities of the leaders. It is common for matters related to young people or women, such as contraception or maternal mortality, to receive less priority than they deserve.

Encourage, organize and participate

It is easy to talk about what is wrong. It is much more difficult to put things right. When the people have decided what the main health problems are, and agreed on their order of importance, a plan of action must be prepared. (See Part IV.)

It is in preparing a plan of action that health workers can help most. From their knowledge and training, they can explain to the people the causes of some problems and how to solve them. For example, if the people are concerned about sickness among children, a health worker can explain various ways of preventing it, such as by protecting water sources, immunizing the children, and improving weaning foods.

The health worker or health team works with the community to put the plan into action, to make changes that will lead to improvement over a period of time.

Inform

Once a plan of action has been proposed, discussed and accepted, the community should be informed of its objectives and of any decisions taken.

It is only when members of the community as well as the health team are aware of these objectives and decisions that their active participation can be sought. If people do not know what is intended, or do not understand why one objective has been proposed instead of another, they are unlikely to do anything to help in achieving it.

The health centre can be one of the various places where team members convey information to the community. It is also a place where the team should use posters, easily understandable graphs, or any other suitable means for informing the public. For instance, it is better to inform the community about practical problems such as garbage and its collection, or latrines, or water supply, than about numbers of gynaecological examinations or urine tests performed.

Summary

- **The purpose of a health team is to work with the community.**
- **Working with the community needs deep understanding of its beliefs, opinions and way of life.**
- **Working with the community means:**
  - **— observing, listening and learning**
  - **— discussing and deciding**
  - **— organizing and participating**
  - **— informing.**

CHAPTER 2
Leading a health team

Learning objectives

After studying this chapter and doing Exercises 14–20 on pages 123–134, the health worker should be able to:

— **ensure that objectives are agreed upon by as many of the people concerned as possible**

— **cooperate with the other members of the health team in setting practical and feasible objectives and targets**

— **understand and apply those factors that motivate people to work**

— **reduce the effects of factors that cause dissatisfaction**

— **decide when, how and to whom to delegate authority and responsibility**

— **choose a style of supervision that suits the health team and the circumstances in which it works.**

This chapter describes how a leader works with a team in community health activities.

2.1 Setting and sharing objectives with the team members

People work well together when they agree with one another and share in the task of setting and achieving the objectives of the whole team. To fulfil the objectives of an organization those who work for the organization should know what its objectives are. People who have not shared in setting objectives or have not been told what these objectives are may waste much effort on activities that do not bring the achievement of objectives any nearer. People who are opposed to the objectives may obstruct the work of the organization. It is very difficult, if not impossible, for real progress to be made in health care without the active cooperation of everyone concerned.

The health worker in charge of a programme and of a health team deals first with people and then with things. People do not give of their best when they are ordered to do things. One of the best ways—perhaps the only way—to ensure that people agree on objectives, and that they are motivated to achieve them, is to make sure that they take part in setting them.

Motivation is an inner impulse that determines what people do and the energy and enthusiasm with which they do it. (See Section 2.2 below.) It is the basis upon which personal decisions are made. People like to make important decisions for themselves. They are much more ready to work towards objectives that they have helped to set than towards objectives set by others.

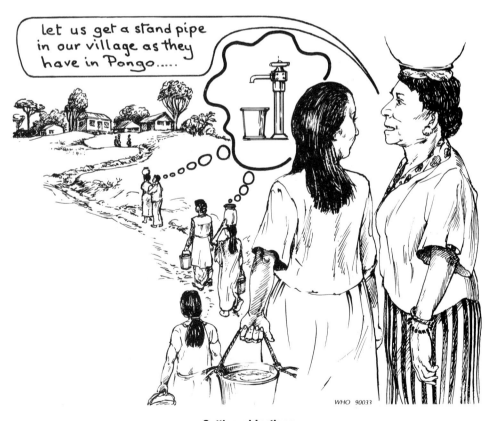

Setting objectives

When local health objectives are being set, various groups of people should be consulted. They include:

— people in the community: interested people from other sectors, e.g. schoolteachers, traditional healers, agricultural extension workers, representatives of workers, leaders (of local authorities, women's groups, etc.)
— patients
— health workers
— the ministry of health (to make sure that local objectives are in agreement with national objectives).

People in the community

It is often very difficult to find out what a community's objectives are, or to what extent a community feels a need for better health or some other social or environmental change that would improve the quality of life. In any community the people should take part in setting their local health objectives; health staff should not be allowed to set them alone. However, some people will try to exert undue influence to further their own interests, and health staff should work to counterbalance such influence by encouraging everyone to contribute equally to objective-setting. It is stated in Part IV that a situation does not become a problem until it is seen to be a problem. Health workers will be aware of many community health problems that are not apparent to the local people. One of their health-education functions is to help the people become aware of these problems. Until the people have this awareness, the health workers will not be able to support them in their efforts to solve the problems.

Patients

Patients demand services. When they have understood their problems and have come to the health worker for a solution, they have a right to be heard. The health needs of a community are often expressed first through the people who are sick. The treatment of sickness may not be the most serious need as the health team sees it but, to gain people's cooperation, the health team must first deal with their expressed needs.

The health workers

One of the purposes of setting objectives is to be able to assess results (see Part IV), and one of the characteristics of objectives is that they should be observable when they have been achieved. Clearly stated objectives encourage health workers to perform their tasks and help them to review and analyse their routine activities. This is why it is important to set objectives that are feasible, and for the health team and the community to reach agreement before final decisions are made.

The ministry of health

National objectives are set by the health ministry and then modified to suit the situation at different levels of the health system. In principle, the ministry of health represents the community as a whole, and sets general health policy. It is a responsibility of the ministry to evaluate the work of its health units and to coordinate their work with that of other government departments, such as agriculture, education, and social welfare.

2.2 Motivating team members

Motivation is an inner impulse that induces a person to act in a certain way. It is a series of internal drives within a person at different levels:

Level 1   To obtain the necessities of life — food, shelter, clothing, rest and safety.

Level 2   To satisfy social needs such as those for companionship, love, and a position of respect.

Level 3   To ensure some degree of personal satisfaction and to pursue ideals. People need to feel reasonably satisfied with themselves, with what they make of their lives and with their talents and abilities.

Using personal motivation to achieve work objectives

A team leader should understand what encourages people to apply their ability and energy to work, and what makes people dissatisfied at work. These two groups of factors may be called *motivators* and *dissatisfiers*, respectively.

The six main *motivators* in work are:

Achievement

Most people like to do things well. They like to succeed. Their satisfaction in success and in getting things done well comes largely from achieving what they expect to be able to achieve and what they aim at achieving. Thus achievement is extremely important to the individual.

Good team leaders help their team members to achieve by giving them clear instructions, suitable training, and the facilities and supplies they need for their work. It often happens that people fail to achieve what they feel they could have done, and they are ready to blame this failure on others. Wise leaders are willing to accept their own share of such blame, but do their best to obtain for their health workers and other people with whom they work whatever is needed to enable them to achieve.

> **HELP PEOPLE TO ACHIEVE WORK OBJECTIVES**

Recognition

Very few people are satisfied with simply knowing in their own minds that they have been successful. Most people like others also to know of their success. An individual can be sure that others know of his or her success only when they respond to the achievements, i.e. acknowledge the success. It should not be hard to praise good work and even to publicize it, but many leaders find it very hard to do so. Perhaps they fear that, if they recognize good work on the part of those whom they lead, their own achievements will be belittled. Lack of recognition can be very discouraging; leaders should be willing to praise others when praise is due.

> **GIVE PRAISE WHEN IT IS DUE**

The work itself

People like to do useful and worthwhile work, helpful to other people and helping themselves achieve their ideals. The staff of an organization like to do work that they can see as contributing to the objectives of the organization.

The appeal of curative medical or nursing work is self-evident. Prevention and health education do not have such obvious appeal, and health workers can find it hard to believe that such dull jobs as accurate record-keeping and inventory control are worth doing.

The good leader will try to keep dull, repetitive tasks to a minimum, and take every opportunity to assure the team members of the value of their work.

> **EXPLAIN THE VALUE OF WORK**

Responsibility

To have responsibility is to be able to accept the consequences, good or bad, of a decision or an action. Most people welcome responsibility; some fear it. Most people like to make decisions about their own lives and to accept responsibility for doing so.

A leader can easily destroy or, at least, reduce staff members' sense of responsibility by making decisions for them. This should be avoided, especially when managing isolated clinics where the staff have to work mostly without direct supervision. The good leader takes the opportunity in such a clinic to increase the staff's sense of responsibility for work rather than diminish it by petty criticisms.

> **HELP OTHERS TAKE RESPONSIBILITY**

Advancement

Advancement is a form of recognition. Recognition without reward is not very convincing. People prefer recognition that comes in a tangible form such as an increase of salary or more responsibility, with freedom to use their own initiative, which leads to job satisfaction.

People's satisfaction often depends as much on what they expect to get as on what they actually get. In acknowledging good work the team leader or supervisor does not make promises of advancement that are impossible to keep. Instead, he or she should encourage people to increase their knowledge and skills so that they become ready for promotion.

> **HELP OTHERS TRAIN FOR PROMOTION**

Self-improvement

People like to become mature, to develop as people. Many make great sacrifices to improve themselves and their families.

Many people want opportunities to discover, develop, master, and use their own abilities to the fullest extent in their work and private lives. Since health workers deal with people, there are endless opportunities for self-improvement at work. Team leaders can help their health workers take such opportunities by providing learning material, by challenging them with questions at work, by helping them set up research projects (which can be very simple), and by giving them high-quality supervision. Given such opportunities to develop, health workers are likely to bring energy and enthusiasm to their work.

> **PROVIDE OPPORTUNITIES FOR PERSONAL DEVELOPMENT**

Objectives and motivation

Objectives are good motivators. A young person who wants to go to college will put great effort into studying, working day and night to achieve this objective. On the other hand, someone whose objective is only to get through school with as little trouble as possible will do as little work as the teachers allow.

Think of the difference between a group of young men running together simply to enjoy themselves and a number of athletes who set out to win a race. The methods they use are similar, but their objectives and results are quite different.

Things that make people displeased with their work are *dissatisfiers* or demotivating factors.

It is easier to be critical than to be creative. It is easier to recognize what makes people dissatisfied at work than to recognize what satisfies them. Obviously, causes of dissatisfaction should be removed, but this may not be enough to take advantage of people's motivations; it may be only the first step.

Six common *causes of dissatisfaction* are:

Inefficient administration

People like to work for an administration that is both efficient and just. Waste of time and other resources irritates them and makes them angry. Even if people do not complain, they dislike being kept waiting. To keep a person waiting is a sign of disrespect; it is the opposite of recognition. Administrators who fail to pay salaries on time, to send transport when it has been arranged, or to distribute supplies cause serious dissatisfaction and discourage their staff.

Incompetent supervision

Supervisors are expected to be technically competent. They must be thoroughly familiar with the details of the work they are supervising. Thus, a midwife's supervisor who cannot help with a difficult diagnosis will lose the midwife's respect.

Poor personal relations

People should be treated fairly. Supervisors who have favourites, or who are dishonest in reporting on the work of the staff, are disliked and the work suffers. People like to be consulted about their work. "He never asks my opinion", "She never consults me", "He never tells me anything" are complaints that indicate poor personal relations.

Poor leadership qualities

People respond much better to example than to exhortation. "Do as I say, not as I do" is a poor method of leading. Leaders have two forms of authority — that of their position and that of their person. Without the personal authority that comes from integrity, fairness and a thorough understanding of the work, the authority of the position of leader will not impress those who are led.

Low pay

The absolute level of salary is less important than its relative level. A salary is satisfactory when the workers get what they expect, what others doing the same sort of work are getting, and what is generally regarded as being fair.

Many people estimate their own value and that of the work they do by the salary they receive. A poor salary has a negative effect. However, a good salary may have only a short-term positive effect. Increases in salary often result in better output and quality of work, but only for a short time.

Bad working conditions

It is normal for health personnel to feel and express dissatisfaction with bad working conditions when these are caused by incompetent or negligent administration and leadership and could be put right. The good leader takes care that conditions of work are such that they permit staff to do their best work. When bad conditions have natural or other causes (e.g. climatic, geographic, economic) outside the control of the administration, the good leader can inspire members of the health team, by example and effort, to do their best in the difficult circumstances.

2.3 Delegating authority and responsibility

The leader of a team is responsible for the work the team undertakes. The leader must make sure that the team has the equipment and resources it needs and that team members are properly trained and able to do the work. The leader is responsible for the team's failures and successes. At the same time, the health workers in the team are responsible for the particular tasks of their individual jobs.

People who can make decisions and see that they are carried out have authority: a health worker who makes decisions about how or where others should work has authority. Authority and responsibility may go together, but they are not the same. People use authority to get the work done for which they are responsible.

One way of using authority is to delegate it. To delegate means to give another person some of one's authority or, in other words, to give another person the power to make decisions.

Delegation has certain *advantages*:

● Delegating some decision-making saves time for other duties.
● When work is spread over a large area, as in rural health work, the health workers on the spot must be able to make decisions according to circumstances.
● Delegation of responsibility saves long delays that occur when awaiting decisions from a central office or other distant authority.
● Health workers who are allowed to make decisions enjoy their work more and become more knowledgeable and skilful.

It also has *disadvantages*:

● If wrong decisions are made, the work may not be done or it may be done less well
● A leader who does not delegate properly may pass all the work on to the team members, leaving very little more to do.
● A leader may delegate decisions to people with insufficient experience.

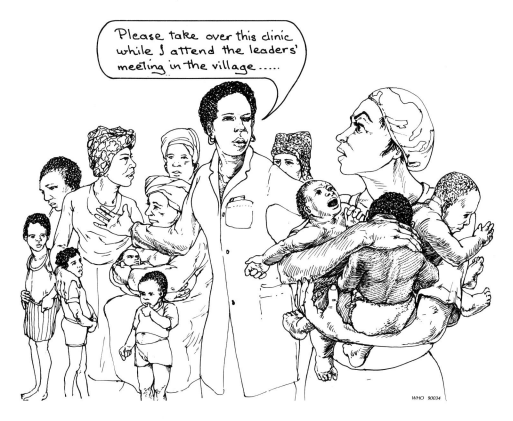

Delegate responsibility properly and for a good reason, and do not cause a subordinate to become overloaded.

Deciding what to delegate and to whom

In deciding what to delegate and to whom, a leader can use a table like the following, listing current tasks in the left-hand column.

Current tasks	Skills used	Health worker who can do this for me *now*	Health worker who could be trained to do this for me
1) Separate weekly meetings with village health workers in three villages 2) 3) 4)	Supervisory Educational Consultative	Medical assistant and auxiliary sanitary worker in turn	

Rules for delegating authority and responsibility

- Be clear about exactly what is delegated.
- Select the person who you are sure can do the work.
- Explain to others that you have delegated work and to whom.
- Do not interfere unless asked to, and be prepared for some mistakes.
- Give support as needed and follow up the progress of work.

2.4 Using different styles of supervision

There are three main styles of supervision: autocratic, anarchic and democratic.

You have probably met supervisors who are very dictatorial, who may say, "Do what you are told, and don't ask questions!". They practise an *autocratic* style of supervision. The health workers have no choices to make and no influence on the type of work that is done. You may have met supervisors who in effect say, "I don't care what you do, so long as you keep out of my way!". This type of supervision can be called *anarchic*. The

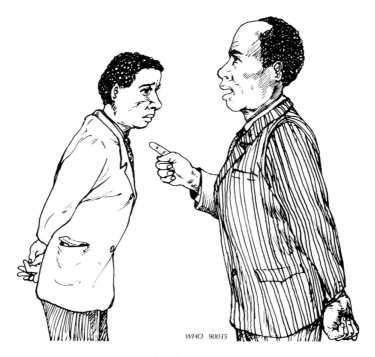

WHO 90035

"Do what I say!"

workers have complete freedom of choice and can do as they like. You may have been fortunate enough to have worked with a supervisor who said to you, "These are the results we have to achieve; this is the job to be done. Let us agree together how best to do it!" This supervisor practises in a *democratic* or consultative way.

Autocratic — Do what I say!
Anarchic — Do what you like!
Democratic — Let us agree on what we are to do.

Autocratic supervision tends to humiliate people and make them irresponsible. It may dry up their initiative. If it is unjustly applied, and it often is, it makes people feel insecure. However, it should be remembered that people need a framework of authority within which to exercise their freedom.

On the whole, democratic supervision helps people to grow, to become responsible for their own work and to show initiative. People like to be consulted. However, instructions must be carried out. Instructions must not become subject to discussion.

Deciding how to supervise

Most people prefer to work under a democratic leadership. This does not mean, however, that the democratic style is always best. The choice of style of supervision depends on the kind of work to be done (job factors) and the kind of people to be supervised (personal factors).

Job factors include:

— the complexity of the job
— the difficulty of the job
— the need for quick decisions
— the need for consistent results
— the need for creative work (new ideas).

Personal factors include:

— the skill, reliability and experience of those who do the work
— their willingness to accept responsibility and to make decisions.

What style should a supervisor adopt? It should not be one that only suits the supervisor's personality and that is not appropriate to the circumstances and needs of the job or to the abilities of the workers. Good supervisors adapt their style to different needs and circumstances.

A consultative, i.e. democratic, style is most suitable:

— for work that demands creativity, e.g. community involvement, research
— with competent and experienced people
— with people who are known to be reliable
— with people who are willing to take responsibility and make decisions.

In certain circumstances supervision must be authoritative, in the sense that instructions cannot be subject to discussion. Such an authoritative style may be used:

— for tasks that demand coordination and consistency, such as dealing with large numbers of people
— for tasks that are governed by strict policies or where immediate action is needed, such as dealing with an emergency or controlling an epidemic
— with people who have little understanding of the goals of the organization that employs them
— with people who have limited skills or experience
— with people who are known to be unreliable.

An autocratic or strongly authoritarian style of supervision can be used only when the staff can be closely supervised and controlled. This is normally not the case in rural health work, especially in isolated health posts. In such circumstances this style of supervision would not be suitable.

The type of supervision practised should be varied to suit the circumstances.

Example: A case-study in supervision

George is the supervisor responsible for leprosy care in Beda District. Some time ago he attended a course in supervision and learned that, to obtain the full cooperation of his staff, he should consult with them and let them contribute to planning.

A few weeks ago George received instructions from the regional leprosy officer that the dose of dapsone was to be changed to 100 mg daily for all adult patients, that treatment was to be continued throughout reactions, and that all new cases were to be given 100 mg of dapsone daily from the day of diagnosis.

This was completely contrary to previous custom. For as long as George could remember, adults received 300 mg of dapsone once a week, treatment began with low doses and built up gradually to the maximum dose of 300 mg a week and was stopped during reactions. George called his dispensary attendants to a meeting to discuss the new drug dosage with them.

When they met, the attendants began to question the wisdom of these new ideas. They said "We have always given patients 300 mg once a week; 100 mg a day is far too much. How do we know that if we give patients 100 mg a day they will take it? Patients cannot come to the dispensaries every day to collect their medicine. We are not even sure that they take 300 mg; some keep the tablets in their mouths and then spit them out and sell them. We have always stopped treatment during reactions. This is the only thing we can do for reactions except to give aspirin. What are we going to do for reactions now? We have been told to build up the dose slowly because many patients are sensitive to dapsone, and a high dose may kill a sensitive patient. Who sent out these instructions? We have never seen him. What does he know about leprosy?" These were only some of the arguments they raised. There seemed to be no end to them.

George said that the instructions had come from the regional leprosy officer, who was an expert in his work. The dispensary attendants would not accept this and the arguments went on for most of the morning. George was unable to answer many of their questions and in his own mind, although he did not say so, he shared their feelings and could agree with much of what they said.

However, George had his instructions. Also, he had met the regional leprosy officer and knew him to be rather hot-tempered. Therefore, to hold his position as supervisor, he would have to put the new instructions into effect. So, after almost two hours of heated discussion, he closed the meeting by saying to the dispensary attendants, "Well, anyway, you must do what you are told. These are the instructions; carry them out."

A discontented group of dispensary attendants dispersed with the new instructions. Later, in his supervisory visits, George found that several of the dispensary attendants continued to give dapsone according to the earlier instructions. One gave 50 mg instead of 100 mg daily, on the grounds that 300 mg divided by 6 gives 50 mg; the patient was therefore getting the same amount as before. A few even continued to give the old treatment, but recorded it as the new treatment in their registers.

Which types of supervision did the superior use in this story?

Considering both the job factors and the personal factors in this story, was the type of supervision suitable?

CHAPTER 3
Organizing health-team activities

Learning objectives

After studying this chapter and doing Exercises 21–31 on pages 134–148, the health worker should be able to:
— **design job descriptions and use them in managing a team**
— **coordinate activities of the team**
— **communicate effectively with the team and the community**
— **prepare and conduct meetings**
— **manage an in-service training system for district health workers.**

The distribution of tasks among the members of a health team is one of a manager's most important functions. When work is distributed unfairly it causes dissatisfaction and sometimes quarrelling. Work should be arranged in such a way that team members use their individual skills and talents. By organization, work can be fairly distributed so that there is no 'overwork' or 'underwork', but all team members carry equal work-loads.

Health tasks are very varied. A nurse, for example, may have to take temperatures, deliver babies, conduct clinics and write reports. This variation in tasks makes organization in health work a challenge to the team leader.

Job descriptions are one means of helping to distribute tasks among the health team.

3.1 Using job descriptions

A job description states:

— the objectives, activities and programmes of the holder of the post concerned

— the authority of the health worker, i.e. the decisions that the health worker is expected to make and has a right to make
— the responsibilities of the health worker, i.e. the expected degree of achievement of tasks and functions.

The purpose of job descriptions is to define exactly for the holders of different posts, their fellow workers and their supervisors:

— what the holders of the posts are expected to do
— what standards they are expected to reach
— to whom they are responsible
— whose work they supervise.

Uses of detailed job descriptions

Job descriptions are a valuable tool for the organization of work.

A job description states clearly what each health worker must do and is expected to achieve.

Job descriptions help prevent arguments between people about who should do what. They help also in the distribution of the equipment needed to do the work.

Job descriptions help prevent gaps and overlaps. It often happens that certain tasks are not done because nobody accepts responsibility for them. These gaps can be prevented by a clear job description for each team member. Without specific job descriptions, two people may think each is responsible for the same job. Such confusion should be avoided.

A job description can show the need for training, for instance if it includes a duty for which the health worker has not been trained or needs further training.

Job descriptions are useful as a basis for evaluating team members' performance. However, they should be interpreted flexibly, as guidelines, rather than too strictly or literally. Thus, team members should be ready to help with one another's work when necessary.

Content of a job description

A job description should be written under specific headings to make sure that it gives all the necessary information.

Job title	This is the standard title for the person doing the work or job, e.g. Nurse/midwife, Grade 2.
Date	The date is included because a job description is not final. People and roles change, and job descriptions should be reviewed and, if necessary, revised at least once a year.
Job summary	This is a brief summary of the main responsibilities of the job.
Duties	This is the central and most important part of the job description. Each duty should be an identifiable entity, a recognizable part of the job-holder's work. Each duty should correspond to one or more programme objectives, which should be listed. The health worker can then see how his or her duties contribute to the improvement of the health of the community.
Relations	These are simple statements concerning:

— the title of the person to whom the job-holder is accountable. For a particular task one person can be responsible to only one superior. However, one person can hold more than one job, and for different jobs may be responsible to different superiors.

— the titles of people supervised by the job-holder. For example, a nurse/midwife may supervise several community nurses in different villages. She is responsible for seeing that they perform their work properly.

Qualifications	A section on qualifications describes the basic training and level of experience required for the job.
Training and development	Every job description should be accompanied by a programme for the further training and development of the person holding the job. This may be, for example, a regular programme of reading or of in-service training, and opportunities to attend professional meetings. Like every other element of the job description, this should be discussed in full and worked out with the job-holder.

Review and appraisal This is a statement describing the process for review and appraisal of the performance of the job-holder. Normally the supervisor is expected to carry out such a review periodically. The review and appraisal statement should state clearly who has this responsibility.

The appraisal may take the form of an annual confidential report written by the supervisor, a simple statement that work is satisfactory, or a recommendation for a change in the duties, or the promotion, of the job-holder.

How to outline duties

The duties of a job are usually determined by:

- *Tradition and training.* These define how similar jobs have been done previously or are done elsewhere. For example, midwives are expected to perform certain duties according to the way they are trained and the way other midwives practise.

- *The interpretation of the person who holds the job.* Experience often leads people to change their way of work or to adapt to new circumstances. For example, a midwife in a village has to work in a different way from a midwife in a large hospital.

  Because rural health work and community work are developing and changing, supervisors and health workers should keep job descriptions under review, so that they remain useful. One way to do this is to get health workers themselves to define their duties.

  A supervisor will find it very useful to ask health workers to list their duties and then to discuss these duties with them; it may be possible to rearrange or reallocate certain duties so that they are performed more efficiently.

- *The requirements of programmes and services.* The objectives and strategies of the services and programmes in which the health workers are employed are the determining factors in the definition of duties and tasks.

JOB DESCRIPTIONS HELP TO GUIDE WORK ORGANIZATION

Example of a job description

Job title	Public Health Nurse for District X.
Date	1 March 1990.
Job summary	To provide, establish and maintain community health through family health care by working with individuals, families and the community, with special emphasis on the welfare of mothers and children.
Duties	1. To plan, organize and conduct the following health services: Maternal and child health Family planning School health Home care Health education of the public.
	2. To supervise the ordering and distribution of equipment and drugs required for the clinics of District X.
	3. To supervise the work of district midwives, community health aides and supporting staff.
	4. To arrange contacts with community groups and actively promote community involvement in the health services.
Qualifications	Registered State Nurse/Midwife with Diploma in Health Education or Public Health.
Development	Prospects of promotion to Senior Public Health Nurse or Regional Health Educator.
Appraisal	Performance appraisal will be based on clinic reports, personal visits and interviews with the community health committees, made by the District Health Officer and the Senior Public Health Nurse. Annual increments and promotion will be dependent on a performance appraisal.

3.2 Using norms and standards

The purpose of *organization* in management is to ensure that implementation achieves set objectives. A job description is an instrument of organization which embodies the principles stated on pages 75 and 76. In particular it states everything a health worker is expected to do as part of the health team so that objectives may be reached.

However, a job description does not say how *much* a health worker must do or how *well*. For this to be done, *norms* and *standards* are established and applied. Norms and standards translate health objectives and targets of health teams to amounts of work and quality of care expected of each health worker. Norms and standards apply to *work*, to *performance*, to *productivity,* and occasionally to *behaviour*.

For instance:

> The number of babies a midwife has delivered in a given period indicates, in a general way, the amount of work she has done (her work output). Comparing this number of babies delivered with the total number of births, in a given area over a given time, gives the health manager a better measure of the midwife's *performance*, as it shows the proportion of the midwifery work in the area which she performed. The *quality* of her performance may be judged in a number of ways — for example, by comparing the incidence of birth complications in the deliveries that she attended with that in the unattended deliveries in the district. To measure the midwife's *productivity* the health manager might relate her work output to a unit of time (a year, a quarter, a month, a week, a day), e.g. three deliveries a week.

The health manager uses norms of work, of performance and of productivity not only to compare achievement with targets, but also to compare health worker with health worker, health centre with health centre and district with district as regards their contributions to the achievement of objectives and targets.

When planners set objectives and targets, they generally have in mind certain norms of work, and of performance and productivity, to ensure that the objectives and targets are realistic. However, health workers cannot be regarded as machines with predetermined production mechanisms; they set their own standards, as part of the process described in Chapter 2, Section 2.1. When this has been done, health workers have many opportunities to assess whether their performance meets agreed norms and is up to standard.

3.3 Coordinating activities

To coordinate activities or groups of activities is to bring them into proper relation with each other so as to ensure that everything that needs to be done is done and that no two people are trying to do the same job.

Coordination is the means of:

— distributing authority;
— providing channels of communication; and
— arranging the work so that
    the right things are done   (what)
    in the right place   (where)
    at the right time   (when)
    in the right way   (how)
    by the right people   (by whom)

When an activity is coordinated, everything works well: a coordinated activity is orderly, harmonious, efficient and successful. When an activity is *not* coordinated, it is liable to fail in its objective: an uncoordinated activity is disorderly, discordant, inefficient and unsuccessful.

An example of poor coordination

A leprosy team arranged to hold a leprosy clinic each month at a certain treatment outpost. When the day arrived for one of these clinics, the medical assistant in charge of the health centre insisted on taking the jeep to the town to obtain supplies. Without their transport the leprosy team could not keep their appointment. Patients waited in vain all day and then went home.

This is *lack of coordination* in the use of transport: the 'when' element was forgotten.

Using organizational principles

To make coordination effective, seven well recognized principles of organization must be applied:

Objective	The objective of each group of tasks must contribute to the objectives of the organization as a whole.
Definition	Each group of tasks must be clearly defined so that everyone knows exactly what the tasks are.
Command	Each group of tasks must have one person in charge, and all concerned must know who this person is.

Responsibility	The person in charge of a team is responsible for the performance of its members.
Authority	Each person responsible for a group of tasks must have authority equal to the responsibility.
Span of control	No person in charge of a group of tasks should be expected to control more than six to ten other people.
Balance	The person in charge of several groups must see that the groups balance. For instance, case-finding must not be so extensive that more cases of a disease are found than can be treated.

A coordinating checklist

A health worker responsible for an action — any action — will find it useful to apply the following checklist:

What is to be done?
Where will the action take place?
When will the action take place?   } Coordinating the activities
What equipment is needed?
How will the action be arranged?

Which members of the health team will take part?
Who outside the health team will take part?   } Coordinating the people
Who will do what?
Who will lead?

Is all necessary information available?   } Communication
Has the information been communicated?

Example: Coordinating group activity health education by using a checklist

WHAT are the objectives of the group learning activity?

To encourage members of a community to participate in promoting health and health care, particularly regarding nutrition of pregnant women and young children. To follow up families who have attended the health centre and, with them, to organize a nutrition programme based on the use of local foods.

Information

The health centre serves five villages. The health workers, in consultation with village leaders, will select one or two women in each village who will be responsible for inviting people to take part in nutrition discussions and demonstrations.

WHEN will the groups meet?

Consult with the community to find out the most convenient time of day, when women are least busy. In the village of Bargong, the women prefer the afternoon. The public health nurse-in-charge discusses the matter with the midwife and a rural health worker. They arrange to visit Bargong every Thursday afternoon for a month. Then they will organize similar meetings the following month in another village.

WHAT equipment and material is needed?

Transport: bicycles for the midwife and the rural health worker.
Local foods to be supplied by the village group.
Flannelgraph to supplement the demonstration.

HOW will the meeting be conducted?

Health workers will discuss child health problems with village women and invite suggestions regarding the content and conduct of the demonstrations.

The women will select the meeting place and between them will provide local foods and cooking utensils.

At the health centre the public health nurse will hold a 'mini-workshop' on nutrition each Monday afternoon with the midwife, the rural health worker, and others who are free to attend.

WHO will take part?

The women in the community, including the young girls; village leaders; the primary health care worker if there is one in the village.

The public health nurse will support and help with the organization from the health centre (supplies, planning the programme, etc.). The midwife will be in charge of the programme at the village, assisted by the rural health worker. The coordination in the village will be done by the leader of the women's group.

Communication

The village woman leader will inform other villagers. The public health nurse will inform the midwife and the rural health worker about the organization and implementation of the programme and will teach and support them as necessary. Other health workers will take part in discussions on the nutrition programme and be invited to suggest other topics for village group meetings. The district health service will be kept fully informed of the programme and its progress.

| COORDINATION HELPS WORK TO PROGRESS SMOOTHLY |

3.4 Communication

Successful teamwork depends upon good relations among team members and especially between the team leader and the other members of the team. It is common experience that personal relations within a team can be difficult. Difficulties are often caused or made worse by poor communication within the team and between the leader and the team members. In the same way, difficult relations may cause, or make worse, poor communication. A team leader should therefore pay special attention to the quality of team relations, and of communication as a means of maintaining good relations.

To encourage communication, the team leader should always observe certain principles:

● All team members should be free to express and explain their views and should be encouraged to do so.
● A message or communication, whether oral or written, should be expressed clearly and in language and terms that can be understood by all concerned.
● Communication has two elements — sending and receiving. When the message that is sent is not received, communication has not taken place. Therefore, the team leader (or other communicator) should always use some means of checking that the intended effect has taken place.
● Conflict or disagreement is normal in human relationships; it should be managed in a way that will achieve constructive results.

How to manage space to assist communication

Always try to arrange rooms, offices, classrooms and other group-education spaces, and tables and seats in such a way that communication takes place most effectively.

● Communication between two people or between one person and a small group

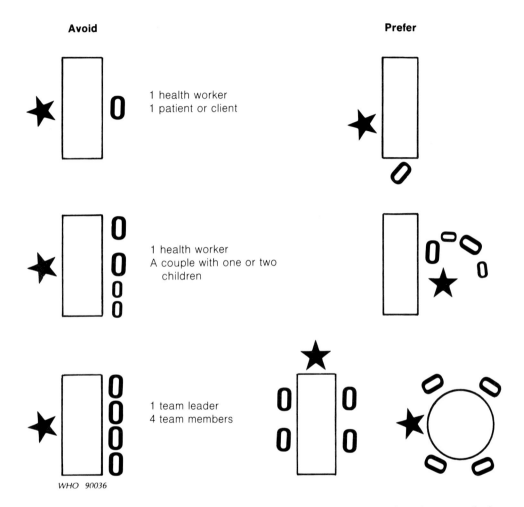

Avoid   **Prefer**

1 health worker
1 patient or client

1 health worker
A couple with one or two
    children

1 team leader
4 team members

WHO 90036

or when the team leader puts another team member in charge of the meeting, e.g. to give the other member an opportunity to learn how to conduct meetings or a training group:

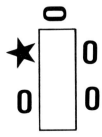

● Communication among small groups (5–10 people)

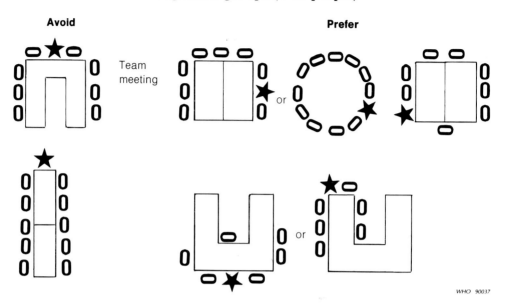

● Communication among larger groups (10–50 people)

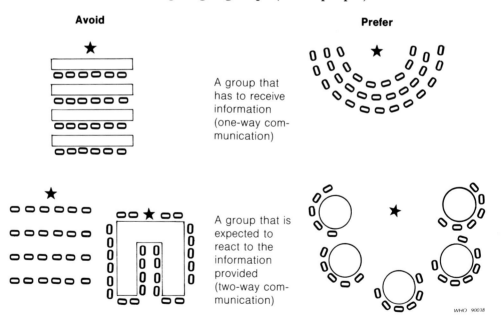

Always remember that:

● In a group of no more than six or seven, everyone can join in a discussion; a big group is therefore better when divided into small groups.

- Tables may hinder communication because of their surface or shape, or the way they are placed. When tables are not necessary (for papers, etc.) do not use them. When you must use them, place them so that the group members can be close to one another. For groups of six or seven, pairs of small tables may be placed next to each other. This arrangement enables several groups to work together in the same room, both as separate small groups and as one large group, as necessary.
- Avoid long and U-shaped tables.
- Do not place tables in such a way as to show or emphasize that certain people have high rank and others low rank, unless you have a valid reason for doing so.

Seating arrangements should reflect the purpose or objective of the meetings or groups. Use such arrangements to make communication easy, if this is important for the purpose or objective. Adapt the seating arrangements to the purpose, not the purpose to the seating arrangements.

Example 1: Communication difficulties between an educated health worker and a villager

The health worker:

- has a scientific attitude towards disease
- uses medical terms
- regards the health centre as an acceptable institution
- thinks of the 45 other people he or she still has to see
- has been educated and trained in the city and may have lost touch with rural life.

The villager:

- has a personal fear of his or her own illness
- does not understand medical terms
- fears hospital because it is an unknown place
- is concerned only to get well
- is a working person with little or no education or experience of life beyond the village.

Example 2: A story about non-communication in management

A medical assistant wakes up one morning and remembers that there is an important meeting of the district council. It is important because it will be discussing a grant to the health centre to build a small local-type kitchen for educating mothers in nutrition. He takes the jeep and goes off to the meeting, only 8 kilometres away.

The senior nurse arrives at the health centre and starts her morning clinic. A young nurse aide asks her to see a mother who arrived in labour during the night.

Finding a prolapsed arm, the senior nurse asks the junior to find the driver to transport the woman urgently to the district hospital. The junior nurse reports that neither the driver nor the jeep can be found. The sweeper is sent to search. The medical assistant's house is locked; his wife has gone to the market. The driver's wife knows only that her husband went to work that morning. The senior nurse tells the woman's relatives to find private transport urgently.

Meanwhile, a large number of patients are waiting outside the medical assistant's door to see him, and another group are waiting in the maternity clinic to see the senior nurse. Two hours have passed but nobody has told them anything. A waiting local shopkeeper is becoming annoyed; he starts shouting abuse. Nobody knows where the medical assistant is. The senior nurse advises all patients who are not very ill to return home. She asks the junior nurse to take her maternity clinic while she sees the remaining patients waiting for the medical assistant. The leader of the Women's Club is waiting in the maternity clinic. She refuses to be examined by the junior nurse and demands the senior nurse. When the senior nurse arrives she explains the situation to the women's leader and the other waiting women. They then calm down and accept the situation, but say "Why didn't you explain this to us before?"

At 2.00 p.m. the district medical officer (DMO) arrives. It is a surprise visit. He had planned to visit during the previous week but had not come. Meanwhile, all the patients who had been collected to see him last week have returned home. Because the medical assistant is absent and there are no special patients to see, the DMO decides to inspect the clinic registers. However, these are in a locked cupboard and nobody knows where the keys are kept. The DMO returns to the district hospital having accomplished nothing.

Example 2 contains several typical instances of lack of communication.

If the medical assistant had left a note to say where he was, the jeep could have been found to take the woman to hospital. If the patients had been told of the situation earlier the non-serious cases need not have waited two hours, the local shopkeeper would not have been antagonized and the women's leader would not have wasted time demanding explanations.

If the DMO had communicated both when he was *not* coming and when he *would be* coming, he could have seen a number of patients with difficult problems who had been waiting for his visit.

The keys to the cupboard containing the clinic registers should have been in the possession of some responsible person, and the rest of the staff should have known who that person was.

3.5 Conducting meetings

Meetings are a necessary part of health work, especially when the work is with rural communities.

Meetings are of many kinds and can have many different purposes. There may be large public meetings, often held in the open air, to encourage people to express their views on a new project or to inform them of, and explain, something new. Small meetings may be held with community leaders to try to identify health problems and needs. There may be meetings with special groups such as patients or mothers for purposes of health education.

There are also regular meetings of the health team. Sometimes there are committee meetings to make decisions on a new project, or educational meetings or discussion groups to learn new skills and new approaches.

Preparing for a meeting

When preparing for a meeting it is useful to check the following items:

— purpose of meeting
— main subject-matter
— type of meeting
— size of meeting
— place, time, and duration of meeting
— who is convening and organizing the meeting
— announcements or information about the meeting.

Purpose

The purpose of the meeting should be very clear. For a formal committee the agenda should state the purpose. However, it is worth writing a brief summary of the purpose, stating what it is hoped to achieve.

Some meetings are called to communicate information, others to exchange views and ideas, and others to make decisions about plans or activities.

Subject matter

If a meeting is to be useful, each person present must have as much information as possible about the subject to be discussed. Also, the facts,

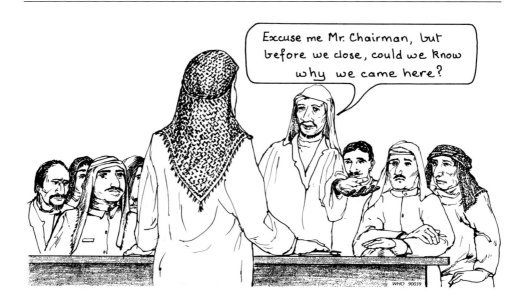

principles or ideas needed as a basis for the discussion must be provided, sometimes before the meeting by means perhaps of a book or a working paper, or at the meeting by a knowledgeable person or by use of a tape-recording or a film. If the subject for discussion is new to several members of the group, someone who has special knowledge of the subject should be asked to give a brief introduction.

Type of meeting

Meetings may be small or large, formal or informal, and open to all or only to members.

Size of the meeting

The size of a meeting largely determines how a subject is discussed, whether everybody takes part, and whether it is easy to reach decisions or take votes.

Two or three people may be enough when the group is meeting to share ideas or for a spontaneous discussion in a search for new ideas. A group of five to seven people is usually large enough to provide a reasonable variety of experience and personalities and, at the same time, enable everyone to participate. As a general rule, for group discussion or training, a group should not exceed ten to twelve people. Even with this number a small subgroup may form and dominate the discussion, while the rest of the group become mere observers.

Large meetings are more useful for communicating information and exchanging views than for discussion or making decisions.

Place and time

The choice of meeting place should avoid the need for most people to come a long way; a hall or open square at the centre of a village is often the best place.

The time chosen for a meeting is very important. For a public meeting, the time must suit the public rather than the organizer. People who work all day prefer evening or weekend meetings.

The convener and organizer

The convener is the person who calls people together for a meeting, and may be the health worker or a community leader or the chairman of the group that is holding the meeting. It must be clearly understood who the convener is.

The organizer, who may be the same person as the convener, or a helper, makes the arrangements, e.g. hires or borrows the meeting-place, informs the members, invites the speakers, and provides information in advance about the meeting.

Announcements or information about the meeting

All those concerned with a meeting should know about it in plenty of time. Notices about a meeting may be in the form of written invitations, but are usually posted on walls and doors in public places such as shops or post offices.

Conducting a meeting

How a meeting is conducted depends on whether it is large or small, formal or informal. The chairman should be someone who can encourage good communication.

In conducting any meeting certain factors must be kept in mind:

Communication

The success of any meeting depends on the quality of communication.

If the purpose is to pass on information or to explain something, speakers should find out whether it has been successful, for example by allowing questions and discussion, which will show whether the subject has been understood.

If the purpose is to seek the views of those present at the meeting, the chairman or secretary should summarize the views expressed, or put them in different words, to obtain agreement about what has been said.

Quarrels and shouting at meetings are unhelpful and are often the result of poor communication. When people understand each other clearly there are fewer disagreements.

> **A GOOD MEETING IS SUCCESSFUL COMMUNICATION**

The role of the chairman

The chairman keeps the meeting to its main purpose, gives everyone a fair chance to take part, controls the timing, and keeps order. There are three simple rules for group meetings:

- There must be no rudeness or personal remarks; no member must ever make another appear foolish.
- The chairman must have the absolute right to control the discussion, to rule out irrelevant remarks, and to bring the proceedings to a stop if necessary.
- The chairman should be able to keep the discussion going when necessary, e.g. by raising questions or new topics. At a small meeting, everyone present should be stimulated to take part. Those who are too talkative should be discouraged from talking too much, and those who are hesitant about joining in should be encouraged.

Controlling the time

Controlling the time that discussions and questions take is an essential part of conducting a meeting. Members' questions and discussions must be kept within a definite time-limit to give everyone a chance to speak. If the subject permits, or if discussion is likely to become lengthy, a definite time-limit should be set for a small meeting, with target times being set at intervals. Using time in this way helps people bring their ideas into focus.

If a decision cannot be reached within the time-limit set, it is advisable to postpone the attempt, thus giving time for further thought or preparation.

Committee meetings

A committee meeting is a special type of meeting. A committee is a group of people appointed by another person or group of people for a special function or to attend to some particular business. There are two main types of committee, advisory and executive, and they may be permanent or temporary.

The *advisory committee* advises an individual or another body that has the power of decision. The *executive committee* has certain powers of decision in its own right.

There are three main reasons for appointing a committee rather than an individual:

— so that responsibility may be shared
— to ensure that a reasonable range of knowledge and opinion is consulted before decisions are reached
— to eliminate bias due to self-interest or individual prejudice in decision making.

Committee rules and procedures

When a committee is appointed, the conditions under which it will operate must be clearly laid down, preferably in writing. They include:

— powers and duties
— membership
— voting rights
— arrangements for meetings
— procedure (how it conducts its business)

Powers and duties. A committee cannot function effectively unless there is an official statement of its powers and duties. These are the equivalent of the authority and responsibility vested in an individual, as described in Chapter 2, Section 2.3.

The power of a committee determines what decisions it can take; the duties of the committee determine what its responsibilities are.

Membership. There must be clearly stated rules for appointing members to a committee, for filling vacancies that may occur, for fixing the duration of membership, and for co-opting members (electing additional members to a committee by votes of existing members).

Voting. The voting rights of committee members, including co-opted members, must be defined.

Arrangements for meetings. The rules should specify how often the committee must meet, the procedure for calling a meeting, and who may call it, and how far in advance notice must be given.

Procedure. There must be agreement on procedure, i.e. how committee business is conducted. This must include a rule that states how decisions are reached, e.g. by simple majority, by two-thirds majority, or unanimously. Decisions are generally reached by majority vote; the chairman does not normally vote, but has a casting vote in the event of a tie.

Sometimes a committee must reach decisions unanimously, but this has the disadvantage that one dissenting member may block the committee's work.

The *chairman* or presiding officer is either appointed by the person or group that sets up the committee or elected by the committee members.

The chairman convenes the committee, decides on the agenda, leads the meeting, and signs the records (i.e. the minutes) of the meetings when they have been approved by the members. He or she calls on members to speak at committee meetings and can in certain circumstances deny a member the right to speak. The chairman also puts motions (i.e. formal proposals) to the committee to be voted on and declares them passed or rejected.

The *secretary* records committee decisions. Like the chairman, the secretary may be appointed by those who set up the committee or elected by the committee members.

The secretary's main task is to make a record of the main events of the meeting, and in particular to record:

— the names of members present
— the names of any visitors

— the names of members who were absent and of those who apologized for their absence
— the exact wording of any decisions taken
— summaries of discussions leading to these decisions
— the date of the next meeting.

In recording discussions it is customary not to record the names of members who made particular points.

The *order of business* is as follows:

> The Chairman calls the meeting to order, i.e. begins the formal business of the meeting, announcing the names of members who have sent apologies for absence, and introduces any new members to the other members. He or she recognizes (i.e. accords notice to) any guests who may be present.

> The secretary reads the minutes (records) of the previous meeting.

> Members may raise questions about the accuracy and completeness of the minutes and propose additions or corrections.

> When all members who wish to do so have commented, the chairman will ask for a proposal (i.e. a motion) to approve the minutes. Someone will propose the motion and another second it. The chairman may then give opportunity for further and final discussion, and if there is no discussion the chairman or another member will 'put the question', at which point a vote is taken. Normally the minutes are approved but slight changes are sometimes made.

> The committee then discusses each succeeding agenda item and makes a decision on each one.

3.6 Training staff

Training is a management responsibility

Management uses staff training as a means of making the best use of the human resources of a health system. The quality of health care, and its equitable distribution in a population, depend greatly upon human resources, i.e. upon the staff employed by the health service, and upon certain other people, who may be trained health workers or workers in other sectors, or members of the public who play different parts in health services.

Training is part of the management of resources. The team manager or leader who wants to have the best possible team of health workers — skilled at their work — uses training to make sure that each member of the team knows and can play her or his part, in order to achieve the goals of the health system, both as an individual and in coordination with the other members of the team. The health manager looks for skills or performance, not merely for team members who may know in theory how a goal is achieved. For this reason, training as a means of solving health problems must be closely related to actual work in the field, and thus to the management or solution of priority health problems.

Human resources are the most expensive form of health resource, which is one reason why management should provide for all health staff to maintain high standards of performance. Part of 'keeping fit' for health work is for the health workers to be satisfied with their work and achievements, as well as with their knowledge and skills. This is another reason for management to use training: it can directly and indirectly strengthen motivation.

Uses and purposes of training

Management uses training:

— to maintain and improve the competence (i.e. the combination of knowledge, skills and attitudes) of the health team for all aspects of its work
— to permit the members of the team to obtain satisfaction from, and therefore maintain a positive attitude towards, their work
— to reduce anxieties or any sense of inadequacy that team members may feel when faced with difficult or unfamiliar problems
— to ensure that the health team as a whole, and its individual members, know what they must achieve and have the abilities to achieve it
— to ensure that the community gets the level of skilled health services that will enable people to lead socially and economically productive lives.

By these means, training of district health staff serves the purposes of:

— improving and maintaining the quality of health care
— extending the scope of health care
— implementing health policy and policy changes
— solving or reducing the health problems of communities.

For primary health care, management uses training especially to equip health teams, including community health workers:

— to cooperate with and support communities in becoming self-reliant in health matters (community participation)
— to coordinate their activities with those of other development workers in the community for improving people's lives and therefore their health (intersectoral action)
— to provide health care services in such ways that all those who need them receive them when they need them, and benefit from them (equitable distribution)
— to make the best and most skilful use of referral systems, by means of which the primary level is supported by the secondary and tertiary levels of the health care system.

Management depends upon well-trained staff

Definitions and principles of management were described in Part I, Chapter 1 as follows:

Getting things done: *Management by objectives* and *Learning from experience.*

Efficient use of resources: *Division of labour.*

Economy of scarce resources: *Substitution of resources.*

Getting people to work harmoniously together to achieve objectives: *Convergence of work* and *Delegation.*

These concepts and principles depend for their application upon adequately trained people, upon management keeping itself informed about the actual and potential skills of health teams, and upon a skilful and continuous use of training.

A systematic strategy

Management may use two complementary approaches to performing its training function:

— a national or district programme or system of continuing education of health personnel
— a system of continuing in-service training for district staff.

Continuing education of health personnel

In principle, continuing education is organized as a system that gives all categories of health personnel the opportunity to continue learning throughout their careers, both for their own professional and career development and for the benefit of health services. It is a means by which health workers adapt their performance to improvements introduced into health services and to health and other developmental changes in society.

To the extent that its main purpose is to improve the performance of health services, continuing education is associated with other aspects of strengthening and maintaining staff morale and productivity, as part of development of human resources. These aspects include opportunities for advancement or promotion and mobility within the services, as well as attention to living and working conditions.

However, most countries do not yet have systems of continuing education that are sufficiently responsive to the needs of the health system. Continuing education is still planned and carried out piecemeal, and is therefore largely ineffective. It is often both irrelevant to the needs of health service and communities and unsuited to rectifying deficiencies in the performance of health workers or to filling gaps in their basic education. In particular, it lacks the essential element of ensuring that health workers can apply the knowledge and skills they may acquire to the solution of problems in actual practice. Nevertheless, many countries have elements of continuing education systems upon which district health management can call for support for district training activities.

A system of continuing in-service training of district health staff

Management is normally concerned with staff who have had at least basic training for their health work before becoming members of district health teams (i.e. pre-service training). The responsibility of management is therefore *in-service* training. The training is *service-related* and *problem-related*, and is part of, or associated with, the system of support and supervision of health workers.

It is a function of district health management to make the district self-reliant for in-service training, but supported when possible and necessary by a national or regional system of continuing education.

In-service training:

— is concerned with district or local health needs

— deals with training needs as they arise or become obvious in individuals and teams
— achieves its objectives mainly in the process of problem-solving in health care and, to a lesser extent, by specially arranged 'off-the-job' training in institutions and elsewhere
— uses health workers' work experiences as opportunities for improving skills and understanding
— supports self-learning by encouraging and helping health workers to improve their knowledge and skills
— deals with learning needs before they arise, by means of continuing, regular programmes of education and training focused on priority health problems.

Assuring competence of health teams

Selection and recruitment of staff

Management is first concerned with competence of health workers at the stage of their selection and recruitment. It must have a clear understanding especially of the skills needed to achieve health care objectives. It selects and recruits those health workers whose skills best suit the needs of the job as defined in an up-to-date and valid job description.

A candidate may be selected who is strong in certain of the needed skills and weak in others. Management may then arrange for such a candidate to be trained either before beginning work or afterwards (in-service), so as to acquire or improve the needed skills, or to develop them from actual problem-solving under supervision in the course of normal work.

Monitoring and assessing the competence and performance of health workers: determining training objectives

In the established and functioning health team, the team leader or manager keeps informed of the competence and level of performance of each member of the team by the monitoring and assessment, or appraisal, of performance (see Part II, Chapter 4 and Part IV, Chapter 3). When deficiencies are found in the performance of staff because of lack of knowledge or skills, or because of negative attitudes that affect the use of knowledge or skills, management takes remedial action. First, it determines as precisely as possible the deficiencies in the competence (knowledge, skills and attitudes) of the health worker. These become the training objectives, or the learning objectives of the health worker.

Management then assesses the health worker's potential for acquiring the knowledge and skills needed or for changing the faulty attitude.

If training is then indicated, management arranges for the necessary training or learning experience to take place, until the staff member is judged to have reached the required level of competence. The performance of the health worker is then assessed to evaluate the effect of training.

Deficiencies in performance may be due primarily to factors over which the health worker may have no control rather than to lack of competence. In such cases a management decision to train a health worker, or a category of health workers, as a remedy or the only remedy, would not be a logical decision. Sometimes it is a supervisor who needs training — in supervisory or communication skills, or in the skills of assessing performance. Sometimes it is management itself that needs more training in certain appropriate skills. The deficiency may be caused by poor motivation, lack of resources, understaffing, overwork, or poor organization of work (health workers being obliged to spend an excessive amount of time on paperwork, for instance).

In-service approaches to training

Management uses several approaches to training at the same time:

— training over a fixed period, e.g. a year, and focused on one or several priority health problems of the community
— dealing with training needs as they arise or become obvious in individuals or teams, or as new and unfamiliar tasks become necessary, or when a problem is not being resolved
— using the health worker's everyday work experiences as opportunities for learning
— a self-learning approach, in which individual health workers are encouraged and helped to improve their own knowledge and skills.

Management establishes and maintains a system of continuing education that incorporates these or similar approaches. The system is organized and managed in such a way that it serves the needs of all health personnel, including community health workers not employed directly by the health services. It may be managed directly by the district health officer or team leader, or indirectly by a training officer accountable to the district health officer or team leader. In a small unit it may be managed as one of the functions of a member of the district health team. The system may be a subsystem of a larger system of continuing education at the national level.

Then, the national system supports the subsystem by making various kinds of educational resources available to it and by arranging, when necessary, for members of health teams to take part in training programmes outside their districts.

Relating the training system to the health care system

The training system of the health centre or the district must be integrated closely with service activities. The function of the training system or subsystem is to support the services, by supplying them with the skilled and motivated workforce they need in order to serve the community's health development needs. Part of this function is the professional development of the health workers, which results in satisfaction and pride in their work and consequently in better service to the community. Another part of this function is to make the health workers skilled and efficient self-learners and to support their self-learning efforts.

Requirements of a district system of in-service training

The in-service training system requires:

— an organization with lines of communication to the health services
— a means of training its manpower in methods of recognizing and analysing health problems to discover their causes and means of solving or reducing them
— the ability to implement solutions to those problems, including the training and development of its human resources
— a means of translating proposed solutions into training objectives and learning objectives, to be followed by active learning
— the ability to distinguish non-remediable causes from causes that are remediable or that may be reduced by the use of available local resources
— the ability to determine those causes that are remediable by training
— the ability to determine which category or categories of health workers need to be trained, and for what skills.

The educational process

When the solution to a priority health problem requires changes in working methods, the health workers concerned will need to learn new skills or change existing skills in order to use the new methods. Management then:

— defines the learning objectives
— organizes the learning experiences that will permit the health workers to achieve the objectives
— provides the conditions in which learning can take place.

Defining learning objectives

A learning objective states what the learner should be able to do as a result of the learning experience. In in-service training designed to result in the reduction of health problems or problems within the health service, the learning objectives are the solutions that have been proposed.

The training system must therefore have a means of determining the most likely effective and possible solutions, given the resources and the skills available, as well as the constraints. Difficult health problems may have several 'causes', according to the points of view of different professions and people, and there are correspondingly different solutions. Training may be one such solution. It is rarely the only solution.

Setting criteria and designing methods for assessing achievement of objectives

Once the learning objectives have been defined, management decides on the level of skill to be attained and on the criteria and methods that will be used to assess the degree to which the skills have been attained. The criteria may be listed in the form of a checklist, which itemizes the different components of complex skills and the required levels of performance. Such a checklist tells both the learner and the trainer the elements of the skill or performance to be acquired. In practice, however, when the objective of training and learning is to solve a health problem, the experienced trainer, supervisor or team leader can judge the adequacy of a health worker's performance and the level of skill achieved or yet to be achieved.

Selecting learning methods

When the learning objectives and the methods of assessing their achievement have been determined, the method of training and of achieving each learning objective or group of objectives is decided. The method must always be appropriate to the objectives. When a skill or a group of skills is the objective, the learning method should permit trainees to practise the different components of the skill, and the skill itself, in realistic circumstances, until they can show, according to the planned method of assessment, that they have acquired it to the required level and can apply it in practice.

Organizing learning experiences

For problem-solving in-service training, management organizes a series of activities, by means of which learners:

— discover what each of them must do in order to solve or reduce the problem (i.e. fully understand the objective)
— become committed to, and motivated for, doing it
— become able to do it in the conditions of practice (which may be very unfavourable)
— become able to apply their new or increased knowledge and skills to a range of similar problems elsewhere and at other times.

The training exercise or series of exercises neeeded to achieve the objectives becomes the course or curriculum or training programme. The methods used will usually require combinations of individual work (individual supervised work and individual work with a trainer or more experienced member of the health team) and group work. Individual work is more efficient for certain objectives and stages of learning, and group work is more suitable and efficient for others. The organizer or trainer or team leader must be sufficiently skilled and experienced in educational methods to decide on the combination of methods to be used, given the nature of the health problem, the training resources, and the conditions in which training and learning take place.

In general, the most effective method involves the solution of priority health or development problems in the course of actual health work. It requires learners to perform, under supervision, the various steps involved in solving actual problems. The solutions to problems, or ways of managing problems, often become apparent only in the course of efforts to solve those problems. Health workers therefore learn problem-solving strategies for dealing with unfamiliar and persistent problems. Management makes available the resources — the supervisors or tutors, the learning aids, the reading material, the equipment, funds, transport, premises, accommodation. In particular, it must provide the conditions that allow the trainees to practise the skills and to use the various learning resources, including means of assessing their own progress in the course of training.

Providing conditions in which active learning can take place

Providing conditions for active learning normally means giving the trainee health workers the opportunity to practise the skills they are to acquire under supervision, until they are able to apply them in the conditions of practice.

Such learning experiences demand active involvement in and commitment to problem-solving, and skilful supervision and support. They also demand that the health workers, usually as part of their normal work, play an active part in identifying and analysing priority health problems and working out the various solutions.

The training is concerned with, and based on, immediate community health problems and on learning needs as perceived by the health workers and their supervisors.

Trainers and health workers use the efforts to solve or reduce priority problems as the learning experiences. This enables the health workers to learn from supervised or guided experience, and enables trainers or team leaders to discover new or different ways of solving problems.

Developing and using training resources

For the purposes of developing and using training resources, management needs skilled staff, for instance a training unit or a training officer, skilled in in-service problem-based training. In a small unit, this may be the manager of the health team or a health worker with part-time training responsibilities who has been trained in the management of such a system.

Management, or the training unit or the health worker responsible for the training must have the means to:

— stay aware of the training resources available in the district and be able to use them skilfully
— have access to and be able to use skilfully a variety of training approaches, learning materials such as manuals, guidelines, textbooks and teaching aids, transport, premises and funds
— be able to call upon and use the resources of a system of continuing education

— use or manage time in a way that permits training to be integrated with health care or health-care development activities; health workers' training takes place in the course of their normal work, but time must also be made available for associated learning experiences outside the work situation.

Reinforcing learning experience with supportive supervision

In order to strengthen and develop the skills they have learned, health workers must use them in actual problem-solving in practice. The function of management in this respect is fulfilled by:

— supportive supervision to help in the integration of the new skills and knowledge with actual practice
— corresponding supervisory skills, adequate time, and transport
— distance learning: this is a means of extending learning from the health centre or educational institution to individual health workers who are at a long distance from the centre and may be alone in their health units or communities; it employs methods based on written, audiovisual or electronic materials that the health workers use in their own time, wherever they are
— arranging for the health workers to meet in groups to share their experiences in applying their skills in the field
— organizing training workshops on specific problems or specific aspects of problems
— arranging for health workers to take part in follow-up meetings and workshops at the health centre.

Evaluation

Evaluation is a judgement of the outcome (in new or improved knowledge, skills and attitudes) and impact (in the solution or reduction of health problems and in better community health) of training and of the process by which outcome and impact have been achieved.

In-service training is designed to improve the quality, scope and coverage of health care and to help in solving or reducing priority health problems. Evaluation of in-service training should therefore be based on measurement or assessment of the extent to which these purposes have been achieved, and the ways in which they have been achieved.

Training efforts are inherently imperfect, and evaluation of training is an essential means of improving them. Evaluation should be able to distinguish between the effects of training and the effects of other activities not connected with training, since improvement in a health worker's performance and in the health of a community may result from factors other than training.

Steps in the educational process

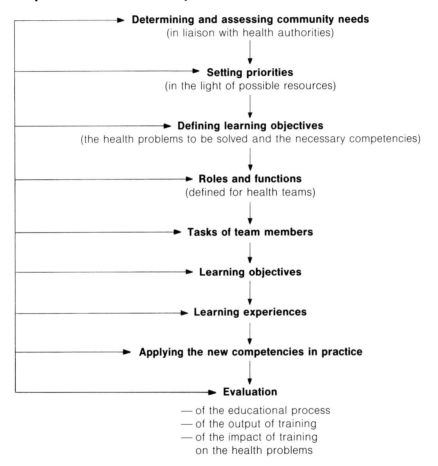

Determining and assessing community needs
(in liaison with health authorities)

↓

Setting priorities
(in the light of possible resources)

↓

Defining learning objectives
(the health problems to be solved and the necessary competencies)

↓

Roles and functions
(defined for health teams)

↓

Tasks of team members

↓

Learning objectives

↓

Learning experiences

↓

Applying the new competencies in practice

↓

Evaluation
— of the educational process
— of the output of training
— of the impact of training
 on the health problems

Summary

- **All health workers need to continue learning.**

- **Supervisors should help in the continuing education of the health team.**

- **Training needs are identified by monitoring and evaluating the performance of the health team.**

- **Learning objectives state what the learners will be able to do as a result of the training.**

- **Training methods depend on the learning objectives. Knowledge and understanding are obtained and improved by practice of the relevant health care skills and by reading, questioning and discussing. Skills are acquired and developed by their repeated practice under supervision until the required level of performance is reached.**

- **Training is evaluated by determining whether, or to what extent, and how efficiently the learning objectives have been achieved.**

- **The training programme or activity is evaluated by its impact on the performance of the learners in dealing with the health problem or health condition for which the training was designed.**

CHAPTER 4

Controlling and assessing the work

When the objectives and duties of a health team have been well planned and the team members have been carefully selected, trained and instructed, control measures can be devised to ensure that the team's work programme proceeds as expected and to help the team and its supervisors maintain the expected amount and quality of work.

4.1 Controlling and maintaining work standards

Control measures guide the work programme and assure certain minimum standards. They are necessary for the following purposes:

— to ensure that work is done according to the objectives set and the activities planned, within the time allotted and with the resources provided

— to enable supervisors to recognize deficiencies in health workers' abilities, knowledge and understanding, and arrange for appropriate training

— to enable supervisors to recognize and reward good work, and to recognize staff suitable for promotion and advanced training
— to enable management to ensure that the resources provided for the work are adequate and are being properly used
— to enable management to determine the causes of work deficiencies.

It is not enough to give health workers instructions and then expect them to carry them out. They need continuing support and encouragement. One way to provide this support is to review their work with them.

Good control should be:

- *Timely*. To maintain work standards, control measures must be taken at the right times.
- *Simple*. Control measures must be simple; otherwise they may take too long to apply and to produce the intended effect.
- *Minimal*. Controls should be as few as possible, i.e. as few as needed to ensure that the work is done and standards are maintained.
- *Flexible*. Controls that are too rigid may be self-defeating: staff will try to evade them.

Methods of control in a work team

Instructions (including job descriptions, objectives and targets)

Instructions must be clear enough to be understood by all concerned, and supervisors must make sure that they are understood. They must be practicable and within the capability of those who are to carry them out; adequate resources to carry them out must be provided. Instructions must be stated in such a way that results can be easily assessed.

Using work schedules

A work schedule shows what a worker or team of workers is to do, and the day and time when it is to be done.

Work schedules are particularly useful for staff who work alone or with only a few other people. They let the health worker in charge of the team know what the team is doing on a particular day or at a particular time, and enable individual health workers to make the best use of their time.

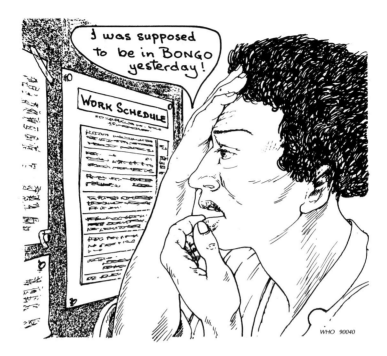

The more specific a work schedule is, the better. Health workers should be required to prepare their own schedules and discuss them with the team leader for inclusion in the overall team schedule. (Detailed guidelines on work schedules are set out in Part III, Chapter 4.)

Time is a most important resource. It cannot be stored or increased; it can only be used productively or wasted. A work schedule helps staff members to use time in the best way, and indicates how long certain tasks take to perform and how much work can be done in a given period of time.

Visits by the supervisor

In supervision, nothing can take the place of visits by the supervisor or team leader to health workers at their place of work. This applies particularly to the management of isolated rural health staff.

Personal visits by the supervisor should help and be welcomed by every worker. The worker should be able to say, "My supervisor knows that I am here and that what I do is important enough for a regular visit to review my work." The personal visit assures health workers that the team leader is someone to whom they can turn for help whenever they need it.

Above all, the visit provides an excellent opportunity for the exchange of ideas and for in-service training. It gives the supervisor a chance to listen to the health workers, to hear about their problems and their ideas for improving their own work, and to assess the degree to which they are aware of the objectives and targets of their health programmes. During the visit, the supervisor should ask the health staff, either individually or as a group:

— what programme objectives they are working towards and what targets they are aiming at;
— whether they consider the objectives practicable, i.e. to say whether the objectives can be achieved in the time allowed and with the allotted resources.

Each visit should have a definite purpose and should be long enough for the supervisor to fulfil that purpose. Visits that are hurried or brief defeat their objectives and leave staff discouraged and disillusioned rather than encouraged.

It is helpful if the supervisor has a checklist of what to look for. This will vary with the nature of the particular facility, department or individual being visited.

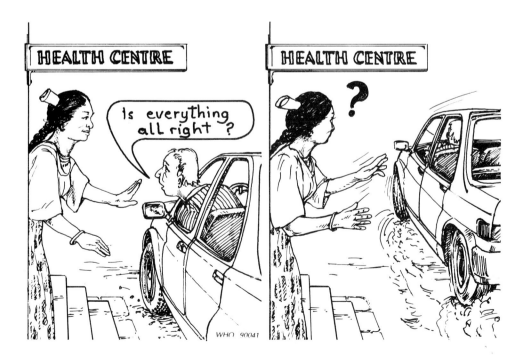

In general, an unannounced visit is not good practice. It suggests to workers that the supervisor does not trust them. Staff should be encouraged to prepare for the supervisor's visit and to think clearly about the sort of help that they want during the visit.

4.2 Assessing work performance

Assessment by a supervisor or team leader determines how close the health team comes to achieving its work targets. It must be based on clear statements of objectives and targets that are:

— relevant to the community's needs
— feasible
— measurable
— known and agreed to by the staff whose performance is being assessed.

The targets may have been presented to the staff in terms of the performance and standards laid down in their job descriptions, or they may be specified in instructions received by workers during training or on-the-job orientation. They may be part of routine instructions or they may be specific targets set by the workers and the supervisor at the beginning of the period that is being assessed.

An important purpose of assessment is to help people discover and make the most of their strengths and correct or minimize their weaknesses. It should reveal — both to the worker and to the supervisor — the worker's potential for growth and development, needs for further training, and the extent to which further training would improve work performance.

Assessment should be continuous. For instance, it is very bad practice to make no performance assessment until the time comes for a supervisor to prepare health workers' annual confidential reports.

The good supervisor will try to see health workers regularly to discuss targets and achievements, successes and failures, strengths and weaknesses. The supervisor must help health workers respond to helpful criticism and improve their performance.

The immediate supervisor, who sees the health worker most often, is the best person to make the performance assessment. It would be unjust for the assessment to be made by someone who sees the health worker only rarely and has little knowledge of his or her work. It would also undermine the supervisor's authority and sense of responsibility for the health worker's performance.

A checklist like the example that follows is often valuable in assessing work performance. (See also The management audit — Part IV, Chapter 3, Section 3.5.)

Example: Checklist for assessing work performance

Code: Y = yes   N = no   P = partly

Name of health worker. . . . .

		Dates				
Work relations	Arrives punctually at work	N				
	Relations with colleagues good	Y				
	Has recently quarrelled	N				
Output	Clinic registers show good attendance	Y				
	Has achieved target in home visits	P				
Skills	Recognizes common illnesses	P				
	Detects at-risk pregnancies	P				
	Sterilization techniques adequate	Y				
	Clinical records clear	Y				
	Supplies and stocks well ordered (systematically arranged)	P				
	Submits reports regularly	N				
Extra	Takes part in staff discussions	Y				
	Volunteers for extra duties	N				

Signature of supervisor. . . . .

Finding work deficiencies

Insufficient training is only *one* reason for poor work performance. There are several others. Many are *not* the fault of the health worker. They include:

— insufficient resources, e.g. lack of drugs
— the health worker lacking a clear job description or clear instructions
— the health worker becoming discouraged by lack of reward or no promotion
— the team members not working well together
— the supervisor not giving enough encouragement
— the health worker having personal worries.

4.3 Records and reports

Records

Records consist of the information kept in the health unit about the work of the unit, health conditions in the community, and individual patients, as well as information on administrative matters such as staff, equipment and supplies.

Records are usually written information kept in notebooks or files; they may also be kept on tapes or be computerized. Records are the administration's 'memory' and an important tool in controlling and assessing work; they are kept to help the supervisor to:

— learn what is taking place
— make effective decisions
— assess progress towards goals.

Records should be accurate, accessible, available when needed, and contain information that is useful to management. Information should not be recorded unless it is known to be accurate and unless there is a use for it.

Before asking health workers to make any records, supervisors should ask themselves the following questions:

● Will this information be used?
● Precisely what useful part will it play in decision-making and evaluation?

- Can this information be collected accurately enough to serve its purpose?
- Will the information be accessible?
- Will it be available at the place and time it is to be used?
- Can the records be stored at reasonable cost?
- Do the records have to be made only because they are part of routine instructions?

At the same time supervisors should make sure that the health centre staff understand the reasons for collecting the information or statistics they have been asked for, and that they are also aware of the uses to which data will be put. Supervisors should discuss with the staff the means of collecting data, and possibly better ways of using them in the work of the health centre or in the community.

Accurate records help team leaders to follow the activities of a programme continuously, according to need.

Special forms, which may differ from country to country, are often prepared and adapted to local circumstances. These forms will help the health staff record the information required, make it easier to standardize the information collected, and save time for all concerned. (See also Part III, Chapter 6.)

Reports

Reports are the information communicated to other levels of the health service. They are also an important management tool for influencing future actions.

The types of report (oral, written, or given by telephone or radio when necessary), their content (statistical information on births, deaths and morbidity, or comments on programme developments or difficulties), and their frequency and use will differ from country to country.

It is often found convenient to have reporting forms printed and distributed in advance to the health units and centres, again with the aim of standardizing information. An example of a village health worker's report form follows.

Example: Village health worker's report form

Health report for the village of ————————————————
Year ———— Month ————————— Name of health worker ————————

1. Number of births during the month:
   - ———— males
   - ———— females
   - ———— stillborn
   - ———— *Total births*

2. Number of deaths during the month:
   - ———— under 5 years old
   - ———— 5 years and over
   - ———— *Total deaths*

3. Number of patients seen during the month:
   - ———— under 5 years old
   - ———— 5 years and over
   - ———— *Total patients seen*

4. Number of patients referred:

5. Type and number of complaints[1] during the month:
   - ———— fever
   - ———— diarrhoea
   - ———— wounds
   - ———— burns
   - ———— malnutrition
   - ———— others

6. Other health activities: ————————————————

7. Health worker's comments: ————————————————

Village Committee's comments: ————————————————
Supervisor's comments: ————————————————

[1] The conditions listed here will vary from place to place.

Health staff must be trained to prepare their reports according to the instructions given by the health services.

Those who make written reports should keep copies of them. Reports then become records. It can be helpful to have reporting forms printed in different colours — one colour to keep at the health unit, another colour for the supervisor, and another for any other interested party.

4.4 Dealing with problems and conflicts

Helping staff to solve personal problems

A good supervisor tries to understand that health staff may have financial problems (for instance, because a landlord has increased the rent), or worries because a child is sick, or a relative has died, or a child has failed an examination. Personal worries are many and varied and may interfere with work. A good supervisor listens sympathetically to personal problems and, whenever possible, tries to help solve them.

A person whose problems are considered with sympathy can work better. One who feels that a supervisor does not care and is unsympathetic may feel resentful and angry, and this may affect the quality of his or her work.

Dealing with disputes

Disputes often occur when people work together in groups and teams. The team leader or supervisor is expected to prevent or settle them.

Preventing disputes

The commonest cause of disputes in a work team is confusion, caused by people having different ideas about what is to be done and how it is to be done. Such disputes can be minimized or prevented by:

— frequent meetings of health-team members
— allowing people to express views openly and letting the whole group decide what should be done
— sharing agreed objectives
— having clear and detailed job descriptions
— having clear instructions and procedures to follow
— distributing tasks fairly
— creating work schedules that distribute work fairly.

A common cause of argument is jealousy and favouritism. A supervisor must behave towards each member of the team with complete fairness and justice, and must never criticize staff in public.

Settling disputes

A serious argument can affect the morale and performance of the whole health team. Arguments must be stopped quickly and the people concerned reconciled. What should the supervisor do in such cases?

First, all the people involved in the argument should be separately interviewed, so that all the relevant facts are known. Second, every effort should be made to discover the true cause of the argument. There is much truth in the saying "It takes two to quarrel"; while more blame may attach

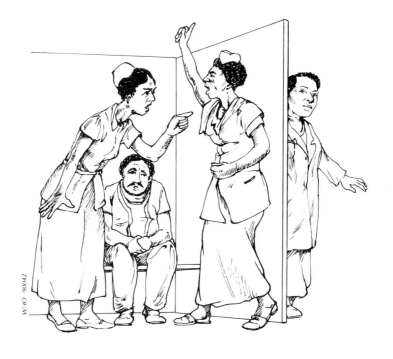

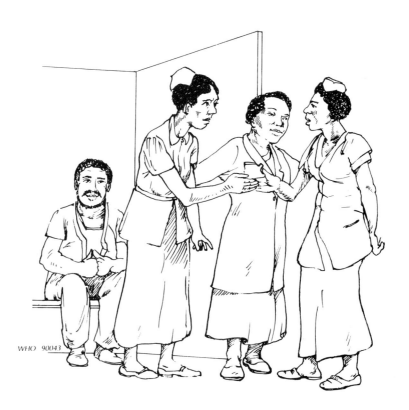

to one side than to the other, there are likely to be faults on both sides. Third, the people involved should be asked — again separately — for their views on how to resolve the argument and about whether they are willing to be reconciled. If a solution can be found that is acceptable to all concerned, productive and friendly working relations can probably be reestablished. If agreement cannot be reached, the best solution is to persuade those involved to 'agree to differ' — to acknowledge the differences in their views but to stop arguing about them.

Summary

- **The supervisor tries to understand the personal problems of health workers**
- **The supervisor tries to prevent quarrelling and bad feeling among members of the health team.**
- **The supervisor tries to reconcile people who quarrel, to bring them together.**
- **Clear instructions and job descriptions, and sympathetic supervision, help to prevent disputes.**

Exercises

Exercise 8 (II.1) Know the community

Objective: To be able to determine the community's opinions and beliefs on health matters.

Individual work

List the items of information you would like to have about the community's opinions and beliefs in order to improve your cooperation with the community.

For each item, decide what you must do to obtain the information.

Decide which members of the health team, of the community, or of the staff of institutions would be best suited to obtaining the information.

Record these data in the table below:

Information needed (opinions and beliefs)	How it may be obtained	Who should obtain it

Group work

Review the list of items of information prepared by the health workers and list all those on which all or most members agree.

Discuss items listed by only a few health workers, seeking an explanation of why they listed them. If the team agrees, add these items to the common list.

Set priorities among the listed items, and review the methods proposed by individual health workers and the activities necessary to obtain each item of information. In each case, discuss the choice of method and select the activities that seem most appropriate and effective.

Review the persons named as best suited to undertake the selected information-gathering activities and agree on who should be asked to take part, from the team, the community or supporting institutions.

Draw up a tentative programme. Record the proceedings of the discussions.

Exercise 9 (II.1) Understand the community

Objective: To improve understanding between the health team and the community.

Individual or group work

For the area for which you are responsible:

— select and list, by name and function, key persons in the community;
— discuss with the team how the various people on your list might contribute to the health activities of the district;
— decide with the team how the listed individuals and groups may be approached and invited or persuaded to participate in a particular health care programme or activity.

Exercise 10 (II.1) Discuss and decide

Objective: To be able to associate with community representatives in joint discussion and decision-making about health matters and programmes.

Individual work

List decisions which you think should be made jointly by the health team and community representatives. For each decision listed, indicate the consultations necessary to reach that decision.

Suggest who in the health team, in the community and in other institutions would be best suited for participating in these consultations and in the decision-making. Record these items in the following table:

Decisions needed about health programme	Methods and activities for reaching decisions	Most suitable people to participate

Group work

Review the lists of decisions prepared by individual health workers. Prepare a common list, including all decisions on which all or most health workers agree. Discuss the others and, if their 'sponsors' are convincing, include them in the common list. Set priorities among important decisions, if possible.

For each decision recorded (taken in order of priority), review the methods proposed for reaching a joint decision, and the preparatory activities discussed. Record the best methods and activities.

Review the list of people suggested as best suited for undertaking the preparatory activities and participating in the decision-making process. After discussing the merits of the various suggestions, record the most suitable names.

Discuss and decide whether to invite those people suggested from the community or institutions to review and discuss your conclusions.

Exercise 11 (II.1) Motivate and participate

Objective: To be able to motivate the health team and the community to participate jointly in health programmes.

Individual work

Study two situations in parallel, and play alternately your own role as health worker and the role of a member of the community. The community member has to decide whether to participate in a health programme that the village health committee and the health team have agreed to implement. Your own position as health worker is that you must decide whether you will take part in a continuing-education programme upon which the district health officer and your team leader have agreed. To find out what motivates the community member and the health worker, write a few sentences explaining or justifying each one's decision to take an active part in the proposed programmes. (*Hint*: such words as hope, wish, desire, expectation, satisfaction, need, ability may be used.)

The community member is *motivated* because:
—
—
—
—
—

The health worker is *motivated* because:
—
—
—
—
—

Then think of all the demotivating factors, i.e. all the arguments that you and the community member may use to decide against participating in the proposed programmes. (*Hint*: such words as difficulties, cost, time, usefulness, waste may be used.)

The community member's *demotivating factors* are:
—
—
—
—
—

The health worker's *demotivating factors* are:
—
—
—
—
—

Group work

Review the list of *motivating* arguments used by the member of the community, note the words most frequently used, and discuss which may be the most powerful motivating factors in the final decision on whether to take part in the health programme. Record these factors in a common list in an agreed order of decreasing importance.

Similarly, review and discuss the *demotivating* factors affecting the community member's decision on whether to take part, and place them in another common list in order of decreasing importance.

Discuss what must be done (not merely what you thought or said) to convince villagers that, on balance, they should decide to take part in the proposed health programme. Write down a list of tasks that each health worker should perform in order to convince different target groups, e.g. heads of families, adolescents, village elders, to take part.

Discuss whether the health workers are adequately skilled for these tasks.

Next, review the list of motivating arguments used by the health worker for participating in a continuing-education programme. Proceed with the same analysis and discussions as for the community member's decision.

Then analyse and discuss the health workers' lists of demotivating factors, using the same approach as above.

Compare the 'for' and 'against' arguments used by members of the community and by health workers, and draw conclusions regarding the similarities and differences in the two groups.

Review the list of tasks necessary to convince target groups in the community that they should take part, and apply it to the group of health workers.

Finally, specify what the team feels it needs to learn to become competent in motivating people, such as resolving to:

— seek guidance on how to acquire such skills, and
— pay particular attention to motivation and demotivation in its work with communities.

Exercise 12 (II.1) Assess

Objective: To be able to assess the relationship between the community and the health team.

Individual work

Consider the relationship between the health team and the community it serves, under the headings:

— communication of information (in both directions)
— cooperation in decision-making
— motivation for achieving shared objectives
— participation in health programmes.

Propose one or more observable *indicators* of the level, or degree, of communication (C), association (A), motivation (M) and participation (P).

C: . . . .

A: . . . .

M: . . . .

P: . . . .

For each indicator, state *who* can observe it and *where*:

C: . . . .

A: . . . .

M: . . . .

P: . . . .

Prepare yourself to discuss this topic, and to present your views on how to assess the relationship between the community and the health team, with the help of the indicators you have proposed.

Group work

Review the indicators that have been proposed for communication, and discuss who should observe the level or degree of communication, and where. Then answer the following questions: Are any of the proposed indicators of communication being used? Being observed? Regularly compared? By whom, and where? What use is made of the findings? Select and retain the most relevant, sensitive and reliable indicators of communication.

In the same way, discuss and select indicators of association in decision-making, of motivation to achieve joint objectives, and of joint participation in priority health programmes.

Exercise 13 (II.1) Community participation

Objective: To be able to involve the community in all phases of a programme.

Individual or group work

Make a survey (in a street, village, or school) to find out whether the community is aware of:

— its priority health problems
— the objectives of the health programme
— the means of achieving the objectives
— what is expected of various members of the community.

Conduct the survey:

— among the population taken at random (as met in the street); and
— among the leaders (or prominent people) of the community.

Exercise 14 (II.2) Setting health-care objectives

Objective: To be able to set, and share, joint objectives for the health team, the community and the health administration.

Individual work

Review your reasons for taking up health work as your profession, list up to ten objectives that you pursue and number them W1 to W10. (*Hint*: think of different kinds of objectives, as described in Part I.)

Then review the list of 'people's' objectives, P1 to P6, below, and add more, up to a total of ten objectives, on the basis of your experience.

Similarly, review and complete the list of objectives of 'health authorities', A1 to A10.

Your objectives	People's objectives	Health authorities' objectives
W1)	P1) Long life	A1) Infant mortality rate down by x points
W2)	P2) Ability to work	A2) Maternal mortality rate down by x points
W3)	P3) Good water	A3) Birth rate down by at least x points
W4)	P4) Good food	A4) Immunization coverage targets: x per thousand
W5)	P5) Services close to home	A5) One physician per x thousand population
W6)	P6) Good quality of care	A6) One hospital bed per x thousand population
W7)	P7) —	A7) —
W8)	P8) —	A8) —
W9)	P9) —	A9) —
W10)	P10) —	A10) —

Then study the entries under "People's objectives" and "Health authorities' objectives". Are they consistent with each other? Do some objectives contradict others — in the same set or in the other set? Do some objectives in one set lack corresponding objectives in the other? Prepare yourself for a group discussion on this topic.

Group work

Review the additional objectives you have proposed on behalf of the 'health authorities' and the 'people'; after a brief discussion agree on how to complete these lists.

Then consider these two sets of objectives. Look for, and note on a board or flipchart, *contradictory* objectives within each set and between the sets, as well as objectives in one set apparently *not supported* by corresponding objectives in the other. At this stage no further discussion is necessary.

Review and compare the objectives proposed by individual health workers. Prepare a common list which should include all those mentioned by a majority of the team members; the list need not be limited to ten objectives. Open the discussion with a search for health workers' objectives that may contradict each other. Note any such objectives and resolve the contradiction through discussion, amendment or withdrawal.

Then search for contradictions between the health workers' objectives and the people's objectives: make a note of these, unless the health workers are willing to amend or withdraw their own objectives. Similarly, search for contradictions between the health workers' and the health authorities' objectives. Make a note of any such contradictory objectives, unless, again, the health workers who proposed them are willing to amend or withdraw them.

Finally, search for the people's or health authorities' objectives that are *not* supported by those of the health workers. Add or amend, as necessary, one or more objectives on the list.

After this discussion, there will undoubtedly remain unsupported or contradictory objectives that cannot be reconciled at this point. Discuss how best to organize negotiations between the three parties to reconcile the three sets of objectives. What should be the ultimate product of these negotiations in order to ensure full endorsement of, and commitment to, the mutually supportive objectives? Record, for later reference, the group's recommendations on this point.

Exercise 15 (II.2) Supervision

Objective: To be able, individually, to express clearly what you expect from supervisors and supervision.

Individual work

Make a short list of what you liked about good supervisors you have had.

—
—
—
—

Write in a few words how you felt about these qualities of a good supervisor.

—

—

—

—

—

Then turn to things you particularly disliked about supervisors you felt to be less good.

—

—

—

—

—

Write in a few words how you felt about poor supervision you have had.

—

—

—

—

—

Prepare yourself to take an active part in a group discussion on your feelings about supervision and the qualities of good supervisors, as well as about the shortcomings supervisors should avoid.

Group work

Review what the health workers have written about their reactions to good supervision, discuss the points needing clarification, and make a common list of the special feelings.

Then review the qualities of a good supervisor as seen by individual health workers and relate each supervisor's qualities to the feelings listed. Prepare a common list of supervisors' qualities.

Go on to review the negative feelings aroused by bad supervision and prepare a common list of these feelings. Then review the health workers' statements about the shortcomings of poor supervisors, and in each case relate these shortcomings to the listed negative feelings. Draw up a common list of undesirable characteristics of supervisors.

Finally, discuss the role that supervisors can play in motivating health workers, and how the demotivating effect of poor supervision can influence the achievement of objectives.

Exercise 16 (II.2) Delegation

Objective: To be able to seek and accept delegation of responsibility and authority.

Individual work

Review all the health care and health promotion activities you carry out currently. You may feel that another health worker could do some of the work for which you are responsible. Name two tasks (say, one in health care and one in health promotion) that might be delegated:

1)
2)

Then state the reasons why delegation might be justified:

Reason for 1)
Reason for 2)

Then list the skills required for performing such tasks:

Skills for 1)
Skills for 2)

Finally, indicate who in the health team currently has the required skills:

For 1)
For 2)

If no one has the necessary skills, what do you suggest?

Now turn to another situation: You have just been told that some management, support and learning tasks will be delegated to you. In each of these fields choose one task you would like to perform:

1) Management task:
2) Support task:
3) Learning task:

State the reasons why you would welcome these new responsibilities:

—

—

—

—

—

Then think of what you should be authorized to do to enable you to perform these tasks well. This may include activities for which you are already authorized.

"I must be authorized to: (for task 1)
                                                        (for task 2)
                                                        (for task 3)"

Decide who in the team can delegate the authority to you. Indicate where you think delegation of responsibility and authority should be recorded so that everyone is clear about it.

Finally, prepare yourself to discuss how best the team might handle questions of delegation in the interest of staff morale.

Group work

Review and list the tasks that individual health workers think could be delegated, and discuss the reasons mentioned for such delegation. Record the reasons in decreasing order of importance (as indicated by the number of people who mentioned them).

Review the health workers' assessment of their own ability to accept such delegation of responsibility, and discuss their assessments.

Then turn to the authority aspect of delegation. Review and list the management, support, and learning tasks that health workers are prepared to have delegated to them.

Discuss the reasons for which the health workers would accept such delegation, and record them in decreasing order of importance (as indicated by the number of health workers who mentioned them).

Review what the health workers have stated they should be authorized to do in order to perform these new tasks well. Agree on a list and record it. Against each of these authorizations, indicate the person who has power to make such authorizations. In case of doubt as to who has such power, make a note for referral to the higher level of administration.

Discuss where delegation of responsibility and of corresponding authority should be recorded, and then how the team should handle delegations (for instance, based on some steps in the present exercise).

Exercise 17 (II.2) Resolving conflict

Objective: To be able to use different ways of resolving conflict.

Individual work

Read the two case studies below and answer the questions that follow each.

Case study 1

You stay at a certain health facility over the weekend and on the morning you are leaving you are told that on the previous day some visitors had insisted on staying in the surgical ward long after visiting hours. The health worker on duty had become very angry with the visitors and had finally shouted at them to get out. He had even threatened to call the police.

The supervisor of the health facility, who had been away for the weekend, is not told of this incident. You are in his office when a local official arrives to make a complaint. He says that the visitors are friends of his and that he thinks the health worker should be punished. The supervisor apologizes profusely to the official and even writes a note of apology for him to take to his friends. This seems to satisfy the official.

You ask the supervisor whether he plans to take any disciplinary action against the health worker; he says that he does not and that he will not raise the matter. By the following morning, however, the health worker has heard from friends in the town of the action taken by the supervisor in apologizing. He feels very strongly that the visitors were at fault and is angry about what the supervisor has done.

1) What do you think of the supervisor's approach to this problem?
2) What might have been a better approach?

3) What action should the supervisor take when he hears of the health worker's feelings about the incident?

Case study 2

A health-centre team leader calls a meeting to consider complaints that have been made about the treatment of pregnant women at the centre since the arrival of two recently qualified midwives.

The women who have complained are not present at the meeting but are represented by the health visitor to whom they have spoken at home. The midwives concerned are not present either; they are represented by the senior midwife. No other staff are present.

The health visitor speaks first and says that several women have complained that the new midwives are too young and too bossy. "They are young enough to be our daughters" said one woman. Another said "They order us about as if we were their children". "They take so long with each case that the clinic does not finish until after dark" said a third woman. "They take blood from us but refuse to give us injections as the old midwives did" said a fourth woman.

The health visitor says she thinks the young midwives are undisciplined and incompetent and that the older midwives (one of whom is her husband's sister) ought not to have been retired.

The senior midwife responds by saying that, in the past two months, the number of women attending antenatal clinics has doubled, partly as a result of a health education programme in the village, but partly because the new midwives are more popular with many of the poorer women. The increased numbers at the clinic have meant that some of the more educated women are being asked to wait longer to be seen and they do not like this. The new midwives are more conscientious about antenatal examinations and this is one reason for the clinics taking longer.

The senior midwife agrees that they lack experience and because of this she has taken responsibility for prescribing treatment herself. She says that she has stopped the practice of giving vitamin B injections because tablets are cheaper and that she no longer gives intramuscular iron injections because the old stock has been used up and the health-centre supervisor has refused to order any more (for reasons the senior midwife does not understand). Finally she says that the matter of discipline of the new midwives is her business and that the health visitor should keep out of it.

1) Was it wise for the supervisor to have invited only the health visitor and the senior midwife to this meeting?
2) Shouldn't the women who made the complaint and the midwives themselves be present?
3) What conflicts are inherent in this situation?
4) What do you see as the causes of the conflicts?
5) What steps can the supervisor now take to reduce these conflicts and to try to repair the damage already done?
6) What other — possibly more effective — approaches to these conflicts might the supervisor have taken?

Group work

Discuss the supervisor's approach, and consider suggestions for possible alternative approaches. What lessons do the case studies hold for the supervisory functions of the team?

Exercise 18 (II.2) Motivation

Objective: To be able to explain your opinions about motivation.

Individual work

Respond to the following statements by marking with a tick (✓) the "Agree" or "Disagree" column. Try to give examples from your own experience to support your answer.

	Agree	Disagree
Most people do not care whether they do good work or not.		
Health-team members give better health care when their work is recognized.		
Health-team members give better health care when they are closely supervised.		
Health-team leaders should try to motivate their team members by giving them responsibility for their own work.		
The importance of good records is so obvious that there is no need to explain the uses of records to health-team members.		
The best way to motivate people is to pay them a higher salary.		
Health-team members should be discouraged from trying to better themselves, because if one member of a team is promoted others will become envious.		
Provided salaries are paid on time, most health-team members will not be concerned about other signs of poor administration such as late deliveries of medicines.		
People work together better when they agree about the goals of the work.		

It does not matter to health-team members if the supervisor has favourites among them.   ———   ————

People do not respect a leader who asks their opinion before making decisions about the work.   ———   ————

People will lose respect for a leader who admits he has made a mistake and changes his decision about an important matter.   ———   ————

Group work

These statements may also be used as a basis for group discussion.

Exercise 19 (II.2) Self-evaluation of leadership

Objective: To be able to express your own ideas about leadership.

Individual or group work

You are asked to give your opinion on each of the following pairs of statements by marking a cross (×) in the appropriate place on the 1-to-5 scale. For instance, in the first statement, if you feel that jobs should be clearly defined and not changed, then put a cross under 1. If you feel that jobs should be flexible and people should always discuss what to do, put a cross under 5. However, if you feel that there are times when no changes are needed but that limits should be set to flexibility, put the cross under 3.

What sort of leadership do you favour?

	1	2	3	4	5	
Jobs should be clearly defined and not changed much.	—	—	—	—	—	Jobs should be flexible and people should discuss what to do.
There should be clear lines of authority, with the person at the top carrying responsibility for all aspects of the work.	—	—	—	—	—	There should be delegation of authority and responsibility to those doing the job.
People work best in order to get more money.	—	—	—	—	—	People work best if they get satisfaction out of their work.
Methods of work ought to be defined by outside experts.	—	—	—	—	—	Methods of work should be established by the group or individual doing the work.
Targets should be set and checked by supervisors.	—	—	—	—	—	Targets should be set and checked by health workers.
Groups and individuals should be given only the information they need to do the job, and no more.	—	—	—	—	—	All team members should have all the information they regard as helpful in their work.

Discussions on what is to be done and how it is to be done should be left entirely to management.	— — — — —	Decisions should be arrived at through group discussions including all health workers.
There should be close supervision, tight controls and well maintained discipline.	— — — — —	There should be little supervision, few controls and a reliance on health workers' self-discipline.
	1 2 3 4 5	

Exercise 20 (II.2) Leadership and motivation

Objective: To be able to improve leadership and increase motivation in the team.

Individual work

Study the diagram below:

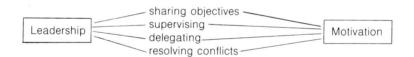

and review the previous exercises relating to Chapter 2. Then list a few suggestions as to what the team should do in order to improve leadership and increase motivation. Proposals should be stated not as general principles but as a series of concrete steps, one leading to the next until desired results are obtained; you should specify who would be involved in each step, and who should be responsible for its implementation. If possible, think of a timetable for implementing the proposed steps. Ideas may be recorded as in the table below:

Steps	Results	People		Timetable
		involved	responsible	
1) 2) etc.				

Group work

Review individual proposals and discuss their merits. Select, first, the desired results; then decide on the steps required to obtain them, set the steps in proper sequence, specify the people involved and responsible, and agree on a calendar for implementation.

Exercise 21 (II.3) Job description

Objective: To be able to write a job description.

Individual work

Using the outlines provided in Parts I (pages 18 and 19) and II (pages 71 and 72), prepare your own job description. (If you have an 'official' job description, do not consult it at this stage.) Make sure you spell out in detail the activities and tasks you must perform in your current job, taking into account any delegated responsibilities.

Then review your official job description, if you have one, and compare it with your own version. Prepare yourself to argue the merits of one version compared with the other in a group discussion.

Group work

Review the job descriptions prepared by individual health workers; compare the two versions (whenever possible) and discuss the advantages of one over the other. Compare the job descriptions of staff with the same designation and amend them as necessary to make them comparable. Compare the job descriptions of staff with different designations and amend them as necessary to make them complementary.

Discuss what to do with the amended job descriptions: for instance, whether to submit them to the next level supervisor with a request that they be considered 'official' revisions.

Exercise 22 (II.3) Norms and standards

Objective: To be able to set your own norms and standards of work performance and productivity.

Individual work

Health care tasks

Review the relevant health objectives and targets for the country as a whole, and derive from them the targets for the district covered by your health team. Note the corresponding tasks in your job description, and calculate the work output you are expected to achieve. For example:

Prenatal care

Objective:	60% coverage of pregnant women in prenatal care (3 visits)
Target:	(District population × birth rate) × 60% = · · · eligible women
Norm per midwife:	(Eligible women × 3 visits) ÷ (number of midwives in district) = · · · annual prenatal consultations per midwife
Average daily output:	(Annual number of prenatal consultations) ÷ (number of workdays) = · · · prenatal consultations per midwife per day.

List the health care tasks for which it should be possible to work out norms as above.
—
—
—
—
—

Now set standards of *quality* of care. The example above contains one such standard: what is that standard? List other possible standards of quality of prenatal care:
—
—
—
—
—

Think of what use you would make of such norms and standards, and prepare yourself to take part in a group discussion on the topic.

Health promotion tasks

List norms and standards that you would apply to the health promotion tasks for which you are responsible:

—

—

—

—

—

Support and management tasks

Suggest possible norms and standards that could be applied to express staff performance in these two areas:

—

—

—

—

Group work

Review the solutions found by the individual health workers, and discuss the terms and calculations involved.

Review the lists of tasks for which similar norms may be established. Make a consolidated list, which will be used in subsequent group discussions.

Review the suggested standards of quality of prenatal care and agree on those that are most relevant, sensitive and reliable. Discuss your ideas about the use (and usefulness) of quantitative and qualitative norms of performance and, if acceptable, arrange to apply such norms in later performance appraisals.

Discuss suggestions for norms and standards that could be applied in the area of health promotion, support and management. Consider whether it would be worth while to appoint a small working group to study how to develop suitable norms and standards in these areas.

Exercise 23 (II.3) Coordination

Objective: To be able to coordinate team activities upon request.

Individual work

You have been asked to coordinate the team's health education campaign. It consists of a series of five health education meetings on the subjects water (W), sanitation (S), nutrition (N), family health (FH), and immunization (I). They are to be held in three villages (each with a population of about 1000) over a three-month period, beginning in about six weeks. The villages, called *A*, *B* and *C*, are each about 20 km from the health centre.

The following activities are involved:

1) Plan the meetings with village committees.
2) Enquire about the special needs of each village in the five subjects.
3) Prepare talks on each subject.
4) Select films and audiovisual materials.
5) Publicize the meetings.
6) Reserve the public address and film van.
7) Conduct the meetings.
8) Evaluate the campaign and report the results.

Assign each of these activities to one responsible person, assisted by resource persons (who may be from among the team, the village leaders, or the district office). In completing the following chart, abbreviations may be used, for instance MO for medical officer, VL for village leader, DHEO for district health education officer, etc.

Activity	Responsible person	Resource persons
1		
2		
3 W		
S		
N		
FH		
I		
4		
5		
6		
7 A		
B		
C		
8		

Study all this information and note whose activities you are expected to coordinate (use the same abbreviations as in the assignment table):

In week   1
In week   5
In week 10
In week 15

In each of these weeks, *what* kind of coordination mechanism would you apply and where:

In week   1
In week   5
In week 10
In week 15

Having completed this, review your activity as a coordinator, and verify that you have all the authority required to fulfil your responsibility. If not, make a note of what additional authority you may require to enable you to function efficiently.

Lastly, try to define the norm of performance you expect to achieve, and consider how your standard should be judged.

Group work

Look for individual suggestions regarding the responsible people and resource persons for each activity, and agree on a complete list of assignments.

Based on the agreed list, discuss whose activities should be coordinated in the four weeks 1, 5, 10 and 15. Given the nature of the activities needing coordination in those weeks, discuss and decide on the most suitable coordination mechanism (*what*). Also, given the nature of the activities and the kind of coordination mechanism, discuss and decide upon the place *where* the coordination should take place.

Discuss any additional authority required by the coordinator, and define, as far as possible, the norms and standards of performance suitable to the coordinating activities.

Exercise 24 (II.3) Communication

Objective: To be able to apply the most efficient and appropriate method of communication in each situation.

Individual work

List the methods of communication you have come across in your professional and private life.

1)   5)
2)   6)
3)   7)
4)   8)

In two or three words record what kind of message was involved in each case (e.g. order, advice, complaint).

1)   5)
2)   6)
3)   7)
4)   8)

Record who was sending the message and who was intended to receive it, in three different instances — choosing different 'senders' and 'receivers' each time.

No.	Sender	Receiver

Then review the following list of situations and choose an appropriate and effective method of communication:

Message	Sender	Receiver	Method (no.)
Request for leave	Staff member	Supervisor	Letter
Technical instruction			
Administrative order			
Sharing objectives			
Consult specialist			
Coordination			
Performance appraisal			
Convey sympathy			
Appreciate good work			
Punish indiscipline			
Advise on use of condom			

Group work

Review the lists of methods prepared by individual health workers. Consolidate and record them in a common list, divided as far as possible into verbal/non-verbal, etc. For each method thus listed, record one example of the kind of message for which it is appropriate, and also indicate and record the corresponding sender and receiver.

Then review the 'message situations' one by one, seeking the ideas of individual health workers as to the appropriate methods for the situation, given the sender(s) and receiver(s) involved. As the need arises, list additional situations, to ensure that each method indicated earlier is represented in the list.

The team should then attempt to identify the necessary skills, attitudes and knowledge required to be able to communicate effectively, i.e. the health workers' perceived needs in the development of some such skills and attitudes and the acquisition of the underlying knowledge. The team may resolve to seek guidance in designing an in-service training programme on this subject.

Exercise 25 (II.3) Meetings

Objective: To prepare the agenda of a meeting.

Individual work

Review the current activities of the health team and list a few decisions that urgently need to be made.
—
—
—
—
—

Judge whether each decision is within the responsibility of the team, and mark with a cross (×) any that is. For any that is not, decide whether the team could contribute to making the decision and mark it × × . Finally, judge whether the team's opinion — even if not asked for — should be made known to decision-makers on issues in which the team has neither a deciding nor a consultative role. Mark it × × × .

Then prepare the agenda (see example below) for a meeting of the team in which all of these urgent matters will be dealt with. Each item on the agenda should clearly state its purpose (reaching a decision, seeking advice, obtaining an agreed opinion), and the necessary documentation (to be provided to the team members in good time). Also for each item name the team member who is to introduce the subject (and who must make preparations to do so). Arrange for the items to be taken in order of priority, and allow sufficient time for each item. State who will be the chairman and the secretary.

AGENDA

For the meeting of the team to be held on . . . .
at . . . .
in . . . .

Item 1:
Item 2:
Item 3:
Item 4:
Item 5:
Any other business:

Signed
(Convenor)

(Secretary)

Group work

Review the 'urgent decisions' mentioned by individual health workers, and list those that were most frequently mentioned. Divide the list into technical, administrative, management, training, etc., decisions. Obtain the views of members on those decisions that are within the team's responsibility to make, those on which it could advise, and those on which it would offer its opinions. Mark these ×, ××, and ×××, respectively.

Then select a few such decisions as agenda items for your next meeting; as far as possible all the various types of decision should be represented. Discuss and decide on the order in which they will appear. For each item, consider the wording suggested by one health worker. Ensure that the person to introduce the item is mentioned, and identify the required documentation. When all items have been drafted, review the agenda as a whole, complete or amend it, and put it on record as an example for reference.

Consider whether to use the agenda as a basis for role-playing in conducting a meeting or in acting as secretary to a meeting.

Exercise 26 (II.3) Conducting a meeting I

Objective: To be able to conduct a meeting.

Individual work

You are the chairman of a committee. How would you deal with the following situations?

1) A non-urgent and fairly minor matter has been rather heatedly discussed for more than 20 minutes and members are still deeply divided on the issue.
2) A member of the committee refuses to yield the floor to another member who wants to speak on the same subject.
3) A member of the committee is habitually late and often wants to re-open an agenda item which was settled before he arrived.
4) The minutes of the previous meeting, as read by the secretary, are disputed by a member. The others have no opinion. The secretary maintains that his record is correct and can show as evidence the notes he made at the time.
5) A member talks at great length about a subject that has nothing to do with the matter being discussed.
6) An important item is scheduled for discussion. Only one member has prepared for the discussion, although a paper on the subject was circulated to all members.

Group work

Review and discuss each situation, and decide what the chairman should do in each case. Record this decision for later reference as an example of management of committee procedure.

Exercise 27 (II.3) Conducting a meeting II

Objective: To be able to act as secretary to meetings.

Individual work

You are the secretary to a committee. How would you deal with the following situations:

1) A motion has been proposed, seconded, and discussed, but no clear decision has been made before the chairman moves on to the next item on the agenda.
2) In your opinion one of the members of the committee is talking too much.
3) A decision has been taken to adopt a motion, but the motion has been modified so much in discussion that you are no longer clear as to exactly what it is.
4) A member disputes your record of a decision taken at the previous meeting, and:
   (a) you have already destroyed the notes you made at that meeting;
   or
   (b) you are embarrassed because your notes on this point were very incomplete (although, before writing the minutes, you had checked the chairman's recollection of what the decision was).

Exercise 28 (II.3) Conducting a meeting III

Objective: To be able to assess how a meeting is conducted.

Individual work

You are to observe a meeting (such as a regular meeting of the staff of the health centre). How will you judge the way in which the meeting has been prepared and is conducted? Under what headings will you assess the effectiveness of the chairman? Write down these headings, and discuss them at the end of the meeting with the chairman, and, if possible, with one or two of the participants.

Exercise 29 (II.3) Learning

Objective: To be able to determine your learning needs.

Individual work

Remember situations in which you felt the need for more knowledge or skill, and record them (marking with a cross (×) any of the following that are relevant and describing other such situations in your own words):

1) Some new responsibility was delegated to you
2) Tasks were being reassigned within the team

3) Visit of a supervisor
4) You applied for promotion to a higher post
5) After your annual performance appraisal
6) You were told of complaints about you from the public
7) You were performing your own self-evaluation
8) In the course of in-service training
9) During negotiations with the local authority
10) When you were asked to act as coordinator for a programme
11) When revising your job description
12) In a meeting for assigning tasks
13) While providing some health care service in the community
14) A serious conflict with a colleague in the team
15)
16)
17)
18)
19)

Count how many times you became aware of a need to learn more. Over how long a period did this happen?

Try to remind yourself of the nature of the learning need you felt. For each applicable situation above, indicate with a cross (×) in the table below whether it concerned health care, health promotion, support activities, management, training, or research.

Situation no.	Health care	Health promotion	Support activities	Management	Training	Research

Review your learning needs and reflect on what happened afterwards; for instances where training followed the awareness of need, circle the cross you have entered in the table. Prepare yourself to discuss this topic in a group.

Group work

Review the situations in which individual health workers became aware of learning needs; establish a common list of the most frequently mentioned situations, in order of decreasing frequency. For each situation, review the nature of the need, and make an entry in the table for the entire team. If any subject is mentioned more than once, enter one cross for every health worker who mentions it.

In the ensuing discussion, consider the situations most likely to reveal learning needs; the most frequently mentioned subjects; the range of subjects about which staff feel the need for more competence; and, finally, the nature and value of any training and learning that occurred. Consider whether the team should resolve to pursue this issue (see next exercise).

Exercise 30 (II.3) Training I

Objective: To be able to formulate learning objectives and select learning methods that correspond to the objectives.

Individual work

You have repeatedly come across the notion of competence, which consists of knowledge, attitudes and skills. Now review the situations listed in the table below, in which various staff members have been put in charge of some activity; in each case consider to what extent the competence required to perform the activity is a matter of knowledge, attitude or skill, and record in the table below:

— 1 for the element you consider *most* important
— 2 for the element you consider important
— 3 for the element you consider *least* important.

Activity	Relative importance of		
	knowledge	attitudes	skills
Sterilization of equipment Organizing supervision activities Coordinating programme activities All public relations with the community Conducting in-service activities			

Choose one of the activities as it applies to yourself and decide:

— what specific knowledge you should acquire,
— what attitudes you should develop, and
— what skills you should master

so that you would feel competent to perform the activity. Record these.

Specific knowledge:

—

—

—

Attitudes:

—

—

—

Skills:

—

—

—

There are many ways of learning. List all those you have come across or know of:

a) e.g. reading   (K)

b)   ( )

c)   ( )

d)   ( )

e)   ( )

etc.

Not all methods are equally suitable for acquiring new knowledge, developing new attitudes, and mastering new skills. Review the learning methods listed above, and record what each method is best suited for in your opinion, using K for knowledge, A for attitudes and S for skills.

Finally, go back to the learning objectives you have set for yourself, and select and record the methods of learning most suitable for acquiring the desired competencies:

—

—

—

—

Group work

Review and discuss the relative importance you have given to the knowledge, attitudes and skills required for each of the activities, and record the group's consensus. Determine the competencies required for performing most kinds of activity for which a health worker may be made responsible.

Then consider the individual learning objectives, one by one. Check that the relative importance accorded to knowledge, attitudes and skills is reflected in the learning objectives. Discuss the relevance and completeness of the individual learning objectives, taking into account that they are precisely tailored to the needs of one person. If two or more health workers have chosen the same situation, compare their objectives and complete or amend them as necessary.

Review the lists of learning methods and record a consolidated list for the whole team, for later reference.

Discuss the suitability of each method for acquiring new knowledge, developing attitudes or mastering skills, and record the majority opinion. (Some methods will be found to have broader scope than others.)

Finally, review the learning methods selected by individual health workers to meet their learning requirements, and discuss the validity of their choices. Record a consolidated statement of learning objectives and of the proposed learning methods, as a possible basis for an in-service training programme for the team.

Exercise 31 (II.3) Training II

Objective: To be able to contribute actively to in-service training activities.

Individual work

Review the statement of learning needs prepared in the previous exercise as it might apply to a team in country X. The proposed learning methods are lecture-seminars followed by individual reading to acquire the necessary knowledge, role-playing sessions followed by group discussions to develop attitudes, and workshop exercises followed by field practice to master the necessary skills.

Decide on visiting lecturers, group discussion leaders and workshop facilitators among health team and district staff who may be requested to contribute to the in-service training programme. Also suggest suitable times for such lectures, group discussions and workshop exercises, over the next three months. Outline a programme including the proposed topics, the suggested responsible people and the schedule. Prepare yourself to discuss your own participation in the programme: for this purpose, extract from this book the references to the topics included in the programme. Prepare your proposal in the table below.

Proposed programme of in-service activities

Learning activity	People		Date and place
	responsible	participating	

Group work

Review the various proposals, discuss a suitable schedule, select suitable lecturers, leaders and facilitators. Assess the interest and commitment of the health workers to in-service training, and discuss whether to submit a similar proposal for in-service training to higher-level supervisors. Delegate to one or two motivated staff the responsibility for preparing such a proposal.

Exercise 32 (II.4) Monitoring of performance

Objective: To be able to monitor your performance.

Individual work

The way in which you do your work is called performance. To monitor performance means to observe and measure certain aspects of the work. Different people will observe and assess different aspects. In this exercise you will look at your performance from your own viewpoint, and try to look at it also from that of the client (patient or community) and the supervisor.

Write down what you would observe and measure in your work performance (e.g. number of outpatients seen):

—

—

—

—

—

Then try to think of how a patient, or the mother of a sick child, would regard your performance, and of how carefully you listen:

—

—

—

—

—

Thirdly, note what aspects of your performance you think your supervisor would be interested in observing and measuring (e.g. punctuality):

—

—

—

—

If you can think of other people whose viewpoints may matter, record them here:

—

—

—

Finally, mark with a cross (×) the aspects of performance for which 'norms and standards' of performance have been set previously.

Group work

Review the aspects of work performance that individuals have indicated they would monitor themselves, and make a consolidated list of all the aspects agreed upon by all or most members of the team. Discuss other aspects and list those on which there is wide agreement. Check how many aspects are the object of some norm or standard, mark them on the list, and discuss what should be done about the others.

Then review the aspects of staff performance that are of interest to the client. Make a common list of all the aspects agreed upon by most or all of the health workers. Discuss the others. Check which aspects are the object of a norm or standard of performance, mark them with a cross, and discuss what to do with the others.

Review and list aspects of concern to supervisors, and mark them with a cross if they are covered by some norm or standard. Discuss what to do about aspects not agreed upon by all the staff or not covered by a norm or standard.

Record a summary of the discussion and consider setting norms and standards for important aspects of staff performance not covered so far, so that as many relevant aspects of performance as possible may be assessed. Discuss whether anyone else, apart from individual health workers, clients, and supervisors, should be taken into account in assessing performance, and, if so, what specific aspects should be monitored.

Exercise 33 (II.4) Assessment of performance

Objective: To be able to discover causes of poor performance.

Individual work

Remember a recent occasion when your performance was assessed as being below the norm or below a set standard. Record what aspect of your performance was being assessed, what the norm or standard was, and who made the assessment:

—

—

—

—

—

Focus on that specific instance of poor performance, and review all the *processes* involved to discover any deficiency that may have caused or contributed to the poor performance. Were there no clearly set targets? Were the norms not clear? Was there some organizational fault (job description not updated, work schedule not finalized, etc.)? Was an important decision not made, or not made at the right time? Underline one or more of the above. Record your comments, if any.

Then consider the *resources* involved. Was there too little staff time available? Was space or equipment inadequate? Was there a shortage of supplies? Was some information lacking, incomplete or misleading? Was money involved? Underline what is relevant, and record your comments.

Then consider the *personal* factors that may have played a part, such as income worries, housing problems, family troubles, illness, conflict with colleagues, a quarrel with clients. Underline any that apply and record your comments.

Can you think of any other factors that might have been contributing to that specific instance of poor performance (e.g. environmental factors)?

The purpose of this exercise is not to find fault with someone else, or excuses for yourself, but to analyse factors that it may be possible to correct or remedy.

Group work

Review one case at a time, record all contributory factors mentioned by the health worker involved, and discuss the relative importance of the factors contributing to inadequate performance. The three most important factors should be marked 1, 2 and 3 in each case.

Agree on how a team, as a regular feature of its activity, might best observe and measure its performance and assess and analyse the causes of poor performance.

Exercise 34 (II.4) Control

Objective: To be able to contribute to the control of factors that cause poor performance.

Individual work

Review the team's record of the previous exercise or, if this is not available, your own individual record. Through this review, you should come to understand the links that exist between the observed deficiencies of process and resources, and personal and other factors, and, more particularly, the links between factors considered most important (marked 1, 2, 3). If such a review suggests some deeper, single cause, this is where correction should take place; each factor is considered by itself, or jointly with others, and suitable corrective action is suggested. Record your suggestions for corrective action in respect of the 'most important' factors:

—

—

—

—

Make sure that the order of priority is clear. Then prepare yourself to take part in a group discussion on how to implement the proposed corrective actions.

Group work

Review the lists of corrective actions proposed by individual health workers, consider fully why such corrective actions are indicated, and estimate how much they may be expected to improve performance. Record a consolidated list for the team as a whole.

Group the proposed corrective actions according to their nature (technical, managerial, communication, training, etc.) and, focusing on one group at a time, decide on:

— who should be the decision-maker to implement the corrective action
— the person(s) who can best prepare the proposal
— the possible obstacles (constraints) to implementing it
— the time-frame for design, decision and implementation
— the cost, if any, of the proposed corrective action.

Record this information for submission to the decision-maker.

Consider the implications for the use of staff time, review and analyse its present use, and set aside time in future staff meetings for this purpose.

Exercise 35 (II.4) Records and reports

Objective: To be able to process the information required to assess staff performance, and to control deficiencies in performance.

Individual work

List below the information requirements for monitoring *and* assessing performance.

—

—

—

—

—

—

Mark with a cross (×) all the information items that are now available to you in existing records or reports. List these records and reports:

—

—

—

—

—

—

Think of possible gaps in information in current records and reports, and prepare yourself to make concrete suggestions for modifying and improving the records and reports in a group discussion.

Group work

Review the reported information requirements, and record them in a consolidated list; mark with a cross (×) those requirements that are currently met. Review and consolidate the list of current records and reports, and determine how such records and reports might be amended to incorporate the information currently missing for monitoring and assessing staff performance. Discuss how to implement these changes.

Exercise 36 (II.4) Supervision

Objective: To be able to prepare a checklist of points to be covered in a supervisory visit.

Individual work

Review the work done and discussed in Exercises 32 (monitoring), 33 (assessment), 34 (control) and 35 (records and reports). In a supervisory visit, performance is monitored, deficiencies are assessed, causes of poor performance are controlled, and some of the findings are recorded and reported. Health workers think of a supervisory visit also as an opportunity to discuss difficulties, to resolve problems, to learn, to communicate and to become motivated. Prepare a checklist of the points you would like to see covered in a supervisory visit so that such a visit leaves a good impression:

—

—

—

—

—

—

At the same time, the health authorities expect the supervisor to be responsible for the effectiveness of the services, the efficiency of the staff, and economy in the use of resources. With this in mind, you may wish to add a few more points to the checklist.

Then think of what you could do to make a supervisory visit a success, and what the supervisor should do.

Group work

Review the lists of points to be covered in a supervisory visit, and prepare a structured, consolidated list for the team as a whole. The list may be divided into categories such as technical issues, organization issues, coordination issues, communication issues, support issues, personal factors, etc.

Check that the list takes into account the supervisor's concern with effectiveness, efficiency and economy.

Discuss how best to organize a supervisory visit so as to deal with all the listed issues — what can be observed on the job, what requires person-to-person discussion, what can be handled in a staff meeting, and what, if anything, requires the participation of community representatives.

Finally, discuss and list the decisions that should be taken in the course of, or following, the supervisory visit. Record the list of decisions required, for review with the supervisor at the next visit.

> **NOW FILL IN**
> **THE EVALUATION SHEET**
> **THAT FOLLOWS**

Evaluation of Part II

On the 0 to 5 scale, mark with a tick (✓) the extent of your agreement with the following statements:

Reading material is:

relevant to my work	0--/--/--/--/--/--5
useful for my work	0--/--/--/--/--/--5
difficult to understand	0--/--/--/--/--/--5
too time-consuming	0--/--/--/--/--/--5

Individual exercises are:

relevant to the subject	0--/--/--/--/--/--5
useful as means of learning	0--/--/--/--/--/--5
difficult to perform	0--/--/--/--/--/--5
too time-consuming	0--/--/--/--/--/--5

Group exercises are:

relevant to the team's work	0--/--/--/--/--/--5
useful for the team's work	0--/--/--/--/--/--5
difficult to perform	0--/--/--/--/--/--5
too time-consuming	0--/--/--/--/--/--5

I have acquired:

new knowledge	0--/--/--/--/--/--5
new attitudes	0--/--/--/--/--/--5
new skills	0--/--/--/--/--/--5

PART III

Managing resources

Introduction

Management is part of the daily activities of every kind of organization.

The preceding chapters discuss concepts of management. However, concepts must be turned into action. All management actions depend upon the objectives they are intended to achieve, and the objectives must therefore be clear. All other aspects of management must be seen in relation to the objectives.

The performance of daily activities requires that many elements — people, time, equipment, material, drugs, etc. — are brought together to achieve an objective, to carry out the work.

The successful performance of activities and the achievement of objectives depend upon the application of knowledge and skills to problem-solving, using all the necessary resources in the most efficient way. Efficiency depends upon how these different elements are managed. For instance, if there is no more ointment because the person responsible did not order it in time, if poor organization of the waiting room means that patients waiting in the treatment room are disturbing the work, if there is no water because the pump has broken down and no steps have been taken to repair it, the work cannot be carried out properly. In terms of management concepts, limitations of this sort will prevent the full attainment of objectives. Proper attention to such details will ensure that, when knowledge and skills are applied to a problem, they will be supported by resources that function and a system or organization that enables the work to run smoothly.

CHAPTER 1

Managing equipment

Learning objectives

After studying this chapter and doing Exercises 37–41 on pages 233–237, the health worker should be able to:

— **explain the difference between the two main types of equipment — expendable and non-expendable**

— **name the four main procedures in the management of equipment**

— **complete an order-form (requisition form) after using the correct catalogue and making a cost-estimate**

— **keep a stock record**

— **record the necessary details when issuing equipment**

— **use an inspection checklist for the control of expendable equipment and maintenance of non-expendable equipment**

— **explain the value and uses of accurate equipment records.**

The two main types of material equipment are known as:

— expendable (also called consumable or recurrent), and
— non-expendable (also called capital or non-recurrent)

Expendable equipment is equipment that is used within a short time, e.g. matches, cotton wool, laboratory stains, paper, disposable syringes.

Non-expendable equipment is equipment that lasts for several years and needs care and maintenance, e.g. microscopes, scalpels, furniture, weighing scales, vehicles, bedpans.

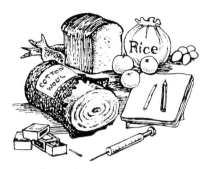

Expendable equipment

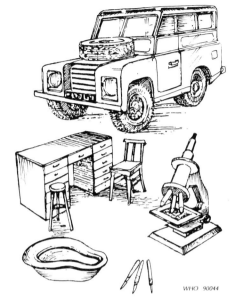

WHO 90044

Non-expendable equipment

The four main procedures in the management of equipment are:

— *ordering* (obtaining equipment from stores or shops)
— *storing* (recording, labelling and holding equipment in a stock or store-room)

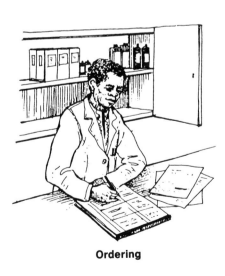

Ordering

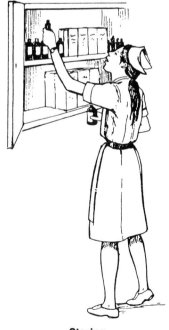

Storing

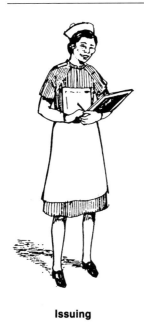

Issuing

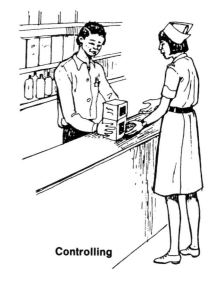

Controlling

WHO 91321

— *issuing* (giving out, recording the issue and the balance of remaining stock, and receiving a signed issue voucher)
— *controlling/maintaining* (controlling expendable equipment, maintaining and repairing non-expendable equipment).

1.1 Ordering equipment

Only some health workers (usually senior staff) are authorized to order equipment; ordering requires the following skills:

— listing requirements, from a knowledge of past use and estimates of present use
— balancing requirements with available resources and making cost-estimates
— use of a catalogue
— completion of order-forms or requisition forms.

Making lists

Several lists of required items should be made, according to the expected place of purchase; for example:

— matches are bought from a local shop
— thermometers are bought from a pharmacy or medical store
— paper is bought from the government office or a stationer.

The exact required type of each item should be written down; for example:

— torch battery, 1.5 volts
— syringe, 5 ml Luer fitting.

The quantity of each item should be estimated, which makes it necessary to know:

— how frequently the order can be placed (purchasing interval); for example:
  kerosene — local purchase, a weekly order;
  thermometers — from a distant store, order every 6 months
— how much is normally used during the purchasing interval; for example, five rolls of cotton wool per month for a treatment room
— whether the amount used is reasonable or whether it seems extravagant or excessive.

The quantity of an item used depends on the number of people using it and can be estimated from experience or by asking an experienced person. Since resources are always limited, consumable items should be used economically.

Balancing needs and resources

Health services all over the world are short of resources. Priorities must therefore be established among needs, and the needs must be balanced against resources (available funds). Sometimes more funds can be obtained, for instance if the budget is increased or a new programme is started. Usually, the amounts or kinds of materials that the health worker wants to order must be reduced until they correspond with the funds available to purchase them. For this, a cost-estimate must be made before completing the order-form.

Making a cost-estimate

The items required, and the quantity, price per unit and total price should be listed in tabular form as shown on the next page.

Items	Quantity	Price per unit ($)	Total price ($)
Thermometers	20	4.50	90.00
Sphygmomanometers	2	65.00	130.00
Sterilizer	1	35.00	35.00
Syringes, 5 ml	10	5.00	50.00
Syringes, 2 ml	40	3.50	140.00
Needles, size 10	200	0.30	60.00
		Total price:	505.00

In the event that less money, say only $435, is available, the list must be revised by reducing or omitting items, until the total matches this amount.

Using a catalogue

A catalogue is a book that contains a list of articles available for purchase from a certain place. It is used whenever things are ordered at a distance. A catalogue may be published by a government store or by a private firm, manufacturer or shop.

Equipment for rural health services is normally obtained through a catalogue order because shops in rural areas are small and do not stock the type of equipment required. Catalogue ordering is also used when purchasing is done through government stores or departments.

A disadvantage of purchasing from a catalogue is that the purchaser does not see the articles being ordered. Often there are several types of the same item (e.g. six different kinds of scalpel or forceps). Articles may also be made of different materials (e.g. kidney dishes in stainless steel, enamel or plastic). The catalogue must therefore be studied with great care and the exact item number, description and price carefully noted.

Completing an order-form or requisition-form

An order-form or requisition-form is usually supplied together with the catalogue. Different stores or firms have their own particular order-forms.

An order-form has a column for each of the following: item reference number, name of article, quantity ordered, price per unit, total price. An example of an order-form is shown below.

Item no.	Name of article	Type	Unit	Quantity	Price per unit	Total

1.2 Storing equipment

Equipment is stored in two places:

— a main or reserve store where stocks are kept but not used
— the place of use, after issue

To store equipment the following skills are necessary:

— recording the receipt of new articles and the issue of articles
— keeping a stock-book or ledger in balance.

Receiving new items of equipment into store

A new item is usually delivered with a document, either an invoice if the item is not yet paid for or a delivery note if payment has been made. Sometimes both papers are delivered. (An invoice is a statement of the cost of the article.)

Invoices and delivery notes must be placed in separate files kept for this purpose and labelled appropriately.

The receipt of the item is then noted in the stock-book or ledger, which usually has a separate page for each item stocked. The record is divided into columns in which are noted:

— the date on which the item was received
— the reference number of the item (from the catalogue) and the place of purchase

— the number of the invoice or the statement of account
— the quantity of items.

Usually there are two ledgers, one for expendable and one for non-expendable equipment.

Keeping a ledger balance

Each item is recorded on a separate page of the ledger. Every time an item is delivered, the quantity received is added to the total in stock. Each time an item is issued, the quantity is subtracted from the total stock. The resulting number is the balance in stock. The following table is an example:

Item	Date	Received from	Invoice	Quantity received	Quantity issued	Balance in stock
Gauze	1/4	GMS[a]	632	10 kg		12 kg
	5/4				2 kg	10 kg
	28/4				4 kg	6 kg

[a] GMS = government medical stores

1.3 Issuing equipment

A health centre may have several sections, such as a maternity ward, a treatment room, a laboratory, a mobile clinic. The health worker in charge of each section is responsible for the equipment in that section. Thus, a maternity nurse may be responsible for weighing-scales, syringes and vaccines, record cards, delivery kits and other apparatus, and a laboratory worker for the microscope, test-tubes, glass slides and stains.

After equipment has been ordered, received, and recorded in the stock-book or ledger, it is issued for use when it is needed. Three paperwork procedures are involved in issuing equipment:

— a ledger record (writing the issue in the stock ledger)
— issue of a voucher which must be signed.
— an inventory record of the section receiving and using the equipment.

Ledger record

When an issue is entered in the stock ledger, the balance of items remaining in stock is calculated by subtracting the quantity issued from the total in stock. When the balance reaches a certain low point, it is time to order new equipment. This is most important: unless issues are recorded in the stock ledger and the balance of stock remaining is calculated, it is very difficult to know when to order more stock.

Issue voucher

The issue voucher is an official form on which are recorded:

— date of issue
— what is issued, in what quantity, and its page number in the ledger
— where it is to be used (section of health centre)
— who is responsible (usually head of section)
— signature of person responsible for its use.

The person who signs the issue voucher takes responsibility for the care of the apparatus or equipment. Issue vouchers must be filed and kept in the store. Duplicate copies are given to the department that receives the equipment.

Inventory

An inventory is a list of items that are kept in a certain place. Each section of a health centre keeps an inventory of its non-expendable equipment.

New equipment issued must be added to the inventory, which is used at intervals to check stocks of equipment in use.

1.4 Controlling and maintaining equipment

Expendable equipment must be controlled to avoid wastage. Non-expendable equipment must be maintained, i.e. kept in good working condition.

To control and maintain equipment the following skills are needed:

— convincing staff that equipment must be cleaned, inspected, and kept in good order, that defects must be reported immediately, and that equipment must always be returned to its correct place after use
— using an inspection checklist and inspection schedule
— detecting discrepancies and explaining them.

Convincing staff of the importance of maintenance

There is no easy way to convince staff of the need to clean equipment and keep it in good condition. The best way is for the supervisor to set a good example and to emphasize that equipment must be cared for:

— to prevent transmission of infection, for instance by dirty instruments
— to keep it in good condition (dirty or damp equipment deteriorates more rapidly than equipment that is kept clean and dry)
— to economize.

It is economical to make the best use of equipment and supplies. Equipment that is well cared for lasts longer; material used correctly is not wasted. (Examples of wasting resources are: using cotton wool for cleaning purposes, not turning lamps down, or not turning off lights when they are not needed.) Equipment should be returned clean and in good order to its correct place after use; in this way it lasts longer and has to be replaced less often.

Inspection checklist

Equipment in a department is inspected by checking what is present and comparing it with the inventory. How often equipment should be checked depends on whether it is consumable or long-lasting and whether it is liable to break down.

Consumable items need to be checked frequently to avoid wastage and extravagance. Long-lasting equipment such as beds, tables and chairs needs to be checked only once a year. Equipment and machinery that is liable to break down (e.g. sphygmomanometers, electric sterilizers, vehicles) need regular and more frequent check-ups.

Inspection is uninteresting work and is therefore often forgotten or overlooked. As a reminder to the supervisor, it is useful to have special set times for inspection, detailed on an inspection schedule.

Detecting and interpreting discrepancies

A 'discrepancy' is a difference between what is reported and what is found, for instance a difference between the amount of something actually used and the amount normally expected to be used, or a difference between the equipment entered on the inventory list and the equipment actually present.

Example 1

The amount of carbol fuchsin stain in a laboratory is the same today as it was three months ago, and there is no record of any having been supplied since that time. This means that the carbol fuchsin has not been used.

It is normally expected that a laboratory in a busy health centre would use carbol fuchsin to stain slides for acid-fast bacilli.

This is a discrepancy in which less has been used than expected.

Explanation. During investigation many reasons might be found for this discrepancy.

- Perhaps no leprosy or tuberculosis patients have been sent for examination. If not, why not?
- The laboratory may have had no acid alcohol and therefore could not use the carbol fuchsin, as both are needed in the stain for acid-fast bacilli.
- There may be a new laboratory assistant who does not know how to perform the stain and is afraid to say so.

Example 2

Twenty 2-ml non-disposable syringes were issued to a mobile clinic. After one month only five remain. This is a discrepancy.

Explanation. Again, there may be many reasons for the discrepancy.

- Perhaps the syringes were badly packed in a box and were broken in transport.
- The missing syringes may have been left behind in a distant clinic.
- Some health workers may have been careless and broken the missing syringes.
- The syringes may have been stolen.

**FIND THE CAUSE OF DISCREPANCIES
AND TAKE APPROPRIATE ACTION**

1.5 The value and use of equipment records

Good management takes care of equipment by:

— instructing and motivating staff to feel responsible for the equipment they use
— ordering supplies when needed
— storing supplies safely
— controlling the use of supplies.

Why is it important to keep accurate records of equipment? Why take the trouble to keep requisition books, stock ledgers, issue vouchers and inventories? Is all the paperwork a waste of time and effort? In fact, there are several good reasons for doing the paperwork:

● Previous order records make subsequent orders, whether the following month or the following year, much quicker and easier. They show suppliers' addresses, item reference numbers, normal quantities required, etc.
● The balance in the stock ledger shows when to order more supplies. This prevents there being long periods without necessary equipment. Being 'out of stock' of equipment reduces the effectiveness of the health services.
● Issue vouchers encourage workers to take responsibility for equipment and can indicate who is accountable for loss or breakage.
● Inventories assist in the rapid checking of equipment in use and in the detection of discrepancies, wastage, extravagance and theft.

In summary, accurate records save time and contribute to the economy, efficiency and smooth functioning of the health service.

KEEP ACCURATE EQUIPMENT RECORDS

CHAPTER 2
Managing drugs

Learning objectives

After studying this chapter and doing Exercises 42–48 on pages 239–246, the health worker should be able to:

— **act responsibly with regard to drugs and set a good example to other staff members**

— **prevent drug wastage**

— **adapt a standard drug list for a health unit**

— **use a decision procedure to make a choice between drugs**

— **on the basis of current use of drugs, estimate drug quantities required**

— **order and stock drugs**

— **issue drugs**

— **establish a method to prevent life-saving drugs from being out of stock**

— **discover and investigate discrepancies in drug usage**

— **prepackage outpatient drugs.**

The use of drugs is only one aspect of a health service but it is one of the most important.

Drugs are important	The management of the drug supply in the health unit is one of the most responsible functions of the health worker.
Drugs are powerful	Drugs must be used with skill, knowledge and accuracy, otherwise they are dangerous.

Drugs are expensive   Wasting or misusing drugs may cause a short-age of supply, with the result that some patients cannot be treated properly.

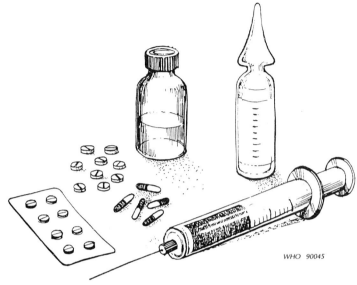

Methods of giving drugs

2.1 Purpose of drug management

The purpose of drug management is to use drugs wisely and avoid wasting them, and therefore to have enough for patients' needs. The following are among the common reasons for drugs, and therefore money, being wasted:

— using too many different drugs on one patient
— using expensive, brand-name drugs when cheaper standard drugs of certified quality would be equally effective and safe
— prescribing drugs before a proper diagnosis has been made, "just to try them"
— using a larger dose than necessary
— giving drugs to patients who have no faith in them and who throw them away or forget to take them
— ordering more drugs than are needed, so that some are retained beyond their expiry date
— not maintaining the refrigerator, so that vaccines and drugs become ineffective
— exposing drugs to damp, heat or light

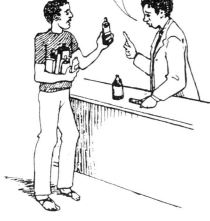

Overprescribing

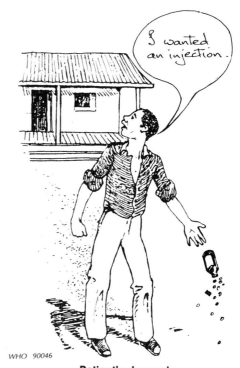

Patient's demand

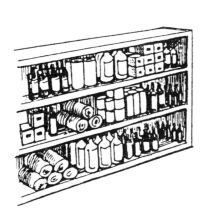

Overstocking

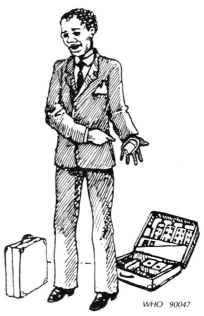

**Prescribing unnecessary
expensive brand-name drugs**

Common causes of drug wastage

— issuing (from store) too many drugs at one time so that they are used extravagantly or even stolen.

Educating staff in the use of drugs

Drugs are important, powerful and expensive. For these reasons, all health workers using drugs should be well informed about them and should show a mature and responsible attitude towards their use.

A health-worker manager can educate staff about drugs in the following ways:

— make notes on the common drugs used, explaining their uses and side-effects, and give copies to all staff
— set out the correct doses of common drugs on wall-boards
— hold staff meetings to discuss causes of drug wastage
— inform all staff about the cost of various drugs
— arrange a lecture/discussion programme and discuss one drug each week at the staff meeting
— put one or more copies of a simple book on pharmacology in the library.

Educating patients about drugs

Patients often take drugs in the wrong way, either reducing the dose to make the treatment last longer or increasing it in the hope of a quicker cure. They take the drugs at the wrong times or forget a dose. Patients on long courses of treatment often stop taking them too soon. This happens because patients do not understand the action of drugs in the body. As a result, they are sometimes not cured and the drugs are wasted.

Health workers should take great care to tell patients how to take their drugs, explaining in a simple way why particular drugs must be taken in particular ways. Thus patients will learn that:

● Each drug has a particular action. A drug that is used for one condition will not help another.
● The size of the dose is very important; if it is too small it acts too weakly to cure the condition, and if it is too large it may poison the patient. Doses for children are smaller than those for adults.
● Treatment must be regular to ensure that the desired level of the drug in the body is maintained.
● The whole course of treatment must be completed; if it is not, the patient may relapse into an even more serious condition than before.

● Drugs must be kept out of the reach of children, who may eat them as sweets and poison themselves.

Special education

Patients with tuberculosis or leprosy who have to take drugs for many months need a great deal of explanation and encouragement. They must continue to take tablets even whey they feel better, in case the disease becomes active again.

2.2 Preparing a standard drugs list

Most health units or sections of a health service have a standard list of the commonly used drugs. Thus, the list for a maternity ward usually includes an analgesic (e.g. pethidine) and a uterine contractant (e.g. ergometrine), and the list for a children's clinic includes a range of vaccines. An example of a standard list for a small dispensary or rural treatment centre is given on pages 177–178.

The standard list is usually prepared by the supervisor or a medical officer and, as far as possible, should be selected from a list of essential drugs established at the national level.[1]

The nature of health work and knowledge about diseases and treatments are constantly changing as new drugs appear. As a result 'standard lists' are often out of date or otherwise inadequate. Standard drug lists may need to be changed for the following reasons:

— diseases are being treated which were not previously treated, or patients who were formerly treated in hospital are now treated as outpatients
— new drugs have become available
— the budget for drugs is no longer sufficient to purchase all the listed drugs and cheaper alternatives are needed.

Changing a standard drug list

To change a standard drug list it is essential to know:

— what diseases and health problems are expected to be treated in the unit

---

[1] See *The use of essential drugs* (fourth report of the WHO Expert Committee), WHO Technical Report Series, No. 796, 1990.

— which drugs are available or could be used for these diseases and health problems
— the comparative effectiveness, convenience, toxicity and cost of alternative drugs
— how to decide between alternatives.

Procedure for modifying a standard drug list

1. Go through the list of conditions treated in the unit in the past six months. Are there any conditions for which no drug is available on the list? If so, add a drug to the list and suggest it to the supervisor.
2. Go through the standard list of drugs and look for any duplications, i.e. two or more drugs serving the same purpose, e.g. aspirin, Aspro, Disprin, sodium salicylate, and paracetamol. If so, choose one drug for each purpose and remove the others from the list.
3. Are there any obsolete drugs, which are never used, e.g. castor oil, chenopodium, arsenical compounds? Sometimes such drugs remain on the shelf or on the list long after they have been replaced by better modern drugs. Remove obsolete and unused drugs from the list and from the shelves.

Deciding between drugs to be included in a standard list

Every decision is based on a comparison of two or more drugs.

If it is difficult to decide between several drugs, make a list of what is needed (the standard requirement) on a table such as those shown in Examples 1 and 2 below. Then list the characteristics of each drug that might be included. Compare each one with the standard requirement, and decide which one best meets the requirements.

Example 1: A mild analgesic for outpatient use

Standard requirements list	Drug 'A'	Drug 'B'
1) Effective	+	+
2) Few adverse effects	Occasional gastric bleeding	—
3) Non-toxic	Low toxicity	More toxic than 'A'
4) Cheap	Very cheap	Expensive

Example 2: A drug for treating large numbers of patients with hookworm infestation in an endemic area

Standard requirements list	mebendazole	pyrantel	levamisole
1) Efficacy	+ + +	+ + +	+ +
2) Treatment course	One dose, or twice daily for 3 days	One dose, or three for heavy infection	One dose
3) Toxicity	None (avoid in early pregnancy)	None	None
4) Cost	Very cheap	Very cheap	Moderate price
5) Administration	Oral	Oral	Oral

Choosing appropriate drugs

When large numbers of patients are being treated for a disease in an endemic area, choose the least expensive drug that is effective, safe and simple to give. Different drugs with a similar effect may vary greatly in price.

When only a few patients are being treated and the disease is uncommon, an expensive drug may be used, despite its high cost.

CHOOSE DRUGS CAREFULLY

Example: A standard drug list for a rural treatment centre

External use

1. Insecticides, antiseptics, soap

   gamma benzene hexachloride (lindane), tincture of iodine, centrimonium bromide, soap

   benzyl benzoate emulsion, benzoic acid+salicylic acid (Whitfield's ointment), zinc oxide ointment, petroleum jelly.

Internal use

2. Antibacterial drugs

   benzylpenicillin (for injection), ampicillin (anhydrous), tetracycline (hydrochloride) or chloramphenicol capsules (depending on local need), sulfadimidine tablets

3. Antiparasitic drugs

   chloroquine (phosphate or sulfate), mebendazole, piperazine (citrate or adipate), metronidazole

4. Antiepileptic drugs

   phenobarbital (tablets)

5. Antiallergics

   chlorphenamine or dexamethasone (tablets)

6. Analgesics/local anaesthetics

   acetylsalicylic acid (aspirin) or paracetamol, lidocaine (hydrochloride)

7. Antianaemia drugs

   ferrous sulfate tablets, folic acid tablets, ferrous salt + folic acid tablets

8. Drugs acting on the respiratory tract

   codeine phosphate, aminophylline tablets

9. Drugs acting on the gastrointestinal tract

   aluminium hydroxide, oral rehydration salts, senna, atropine tablets

10. Drugs used for mental disorders

    chlorpromazine tablets

11. Drugs for the eye

    tetracycline eye ointment

12. Drugs used under supervision for patients referred from hospital with doctor's prescription for tuberculosis or leprosy

    isoniazid, streptomycin (injection), dapsone

13. Vitamins

    retinol (tablets and capsules), others according to local needs

Note: In some cases it may be necessary to stock a wider range of drugs for patients referred from a hospital with a doctor's prescription for e.g. digoxin, phenytoin, hydralazine or reserpine. Similarly, it may be necessary to stock some vaccines and sera.

2.3 Estimating drug requirements: ordering and stocking drugs

Calculating drug requirements

Ordering more drugs than are needed causes wastage, as some may remain unused after their expiry date. Ordering fewer drugs than needed results in shortage, and patients suffer because they cannot be treated. It is therefore essential to estimate approximately how much is needed of each drug. This may be done either on the basis of previous experience in the health centre or by calculation.

Formula for calculation

| Total dose of average course of drug | × | Usual number of patients treated with the drug within the purchasing interval |

The purchasing interval is the time between the arrival of successive drug orders, usually three or six months.

The number of patients treated with the drug or suffering from the disease for which the drug is used is calculated from clinic records or registers.

Example: How much aspirin is needed?

Suppose an average of ten patients a day are prescribed aspirin. The average course of aspirin is two tablets three times daily, i.e. six tablets daily. The purchasing interval is three months (about 90 days).

Then, applying the formula:

Aspirin needed = total dose of average × number of patients treated
course of aspirin in purchasing interval

= 6 (tablets) × 10 (patients) × 90 (days)

= 5400 aspirin tablets needed every three months

If the aspirin is supplied in bottles containing 1000 tablets, five or six bottles should be ordered every three months.

When needs exceed the drug budget

Very often a disease may be so common, or a drug so expensive, that the one disease or one drug alone would use up the whole drug budget. This can be the case with, for instance, gonorrhoea or schistosomiasis, in certain areas. If all patients with gonorrhoea are treated with a full course of penicillin (4.8 million units per patient) there might be no money left to provide penicillin for any other disease or to buy any other drugs.

This presents a very difficult management problem, forcing a health worker to choose which patients and which conditions to treat.

In solving this problem it may help to establish criteria (standards) for treatment. In certain circumstances, for example, 'age' may be such a criterion. In some countries, age determines which patients will be treated by renal dialysis because there are too few dialysis machines to treat all the patients who need the treatment. In some poor countries where many pregnant women suffer from anaemia a limit is set for treatment with iron and folic acid: only women with a haemoglobin level of less than 70 g/litre (7 g/100 ml) are given this treatment.

Other possible criteria for deciding which patients or conditions to treat are the following:

- *Response to treatment.* Has the patient a good chance of recovery if given the treatment? For example, some health centres treat only the acute form of gonorrhoea because it responds much better than the chronic form.

- *Risk of recurrence.* Will the patient get this disease again after being treated? For example, where treatment for schistosomiasis or hookworm is proposed, immediate reinfection is likely unless there is also substantial improvement of the environment.

- *Chronic conditions.* Will the patient need to receive treatment for many years? Patients with complaints such as hypertension, epilepsy or arthritis may need treatment for many years, and a careful choice must therefore be made of which drugs to use for maintenance (e.g. methyl-dopa costs about ten times more than reserpine).

Ordering drugs

The same procedures should be followed as for ordering equipment (see Section 1.1), i.e. requirements should be listed (using a modified standard list, see Section 2.2 above). The exact type required should be stated.

Non-brand-name drugs should always be ordered *when you are satisfied that they are effective and safe*; they are generally cheaper.

The quantity required, dosage form and strength (see Section 2.4 below) should be stated, a cost-estimate (see Chapter 1, pages 163–164) made, and the order-form (requisition form) completed.

Ordering drugs by non-brand names

Many drugs have internationally agreed non-brand names — the international nonproprietary (generic) names (INN).

Brand names are given to drugs by manufacturers. The same drug may appear under many different brand names and be sold at many different prices.

Drugs should be ordered whenever possible by their international non-proprietary names, making sure that the supplier provides the cheapest form available, provided that it is certified or known to be effective and safe and that it is simple to give or take.

Note: In many developing countries large numbers of spurious (false), useless and even dangerous generic preparations are available, which may be bought cheaply and without prescription.

WHO has instituted a Certification Scheme on the Quality of Pharmaceutical Products, in which most countries participate. In these countries the authority that controls importation will know which generic preparations are safe to use.

Stocking drugs

Orderly stocking is an essential part of drug management. Drugs received are recorded in a stock ledger or on stock cards. Exactly the same procedure is used as that explained in Chapter 1, Section 1.2.

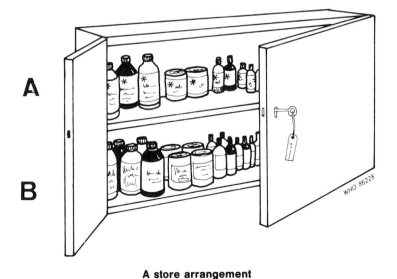

A store arrangement

Note: Shelf A should be used first. The stars show drugs with expiry dates in the current year.

Storing drugs

Most drugs must be kept dry, cool and away from light. A cupboard is best for these conditions. When possible, tablets should be kept in airtight tins and screw-top jars.

Each bottle or tin must be clearly labelled.

A red star or similar mark should be placed on the labels of all bottles or tins with an expiry date in the current year. These containers should be used first.

Dangerous drugs must be kept in a locked cupboard with a special issuing register.

Stock-card system

A stock-card system is sometimes used instead of a stock ledger. It works in the same way as a stock ledger, i.e. a balance is kept by adding items received and subtracting those issued. In the stock ledger each item has a separate page in the book, but in the stock-card system each item is written on a separate card.

In the case of drugs, the card relating to each particular item can be pinned to the shelf next to the drug stock to which it refers. This is a very convenient method for recording issues, particularly if issues are made frequently.

Example: Stock card recording a weekly issue of penicillin

Item: PROCAINE BENZYLPENICILLIN FORTIFIED					
Date	From or to:	Received	Issued	Balance	Remarks
8.11	General medical stores	8000 vials*		10 vials 8010	Expiry: Jan. 1995
10.11	Outpatient department (OPD)		500 vials		
10.11	Maternal and child health (MCH) centre		120	7390	
17.11	OPD		820		
17.11	MCH centre		130	6440	
24.11	OPD		960		
24.11	MCH centre		125	5355	

* 6-monthly order

Study this stock card and try to answer the following questions:

- How long must 8000 vials of penicillin last?
- How much penicillin should be issued each month, to prevent its going out of stock?
- In the three weeks of issue recorded, how much penicillin has been issued?
- Is the rate of consumption (drug use) too high, too low, or just right?
- Which of the two departments, MCH or OPD, would you question about its penicillin use?
- Explain how you would deal with discrepancies you have discovered on this card.

2.4 Issuing and controlling the use of drugs

Drugs are issued, from a locked store or store cupboard, by the person in charge of the drug stock to the section using the drugs. Drugs are issued regularly and in known quantities; this permits monitoring (observation) and control of drug usage.

The frequency of drug issue depends on the circumstances and the type of drug. For example, an infrequently used drug, such as niclosamide for tapeworm, may be issued every six months. Drugs in constant use, such as aspirin or antibiotics, are best issued weekly or monthly. Drugs on the 'dangerous drugs' list are controlled by special laws and are issued only as prescribed for the individual patient.

Each issue of a drug is recorded on the appropriate stock card; the balance remaining is then calculated on the card and checked against what remains on the shelf.

Monitoring drug issues in this way enables the health worker to:

— notice when stocks need re-ordering
— check drug use against patient treatment
— become rapidly aware of discrepancies in drug treatment
— check changes in drug use in different sections of the health unit.

Discrepancies in drug usage are identified in the same way as discrepancies in equipment stocks. The amount of drug expected to be used is compared with the amount actually used. If there is a significant difference, this is a discrepancy.

The amount of a drug expected to be used can be estimated by applying the formula explained in Section 2.3. When one drug is used for several diseases, a total figure for expected use must be estimated.

The amount of a drug actually issued is calculated from the issue records or stock cards.

Investigating discrepancies takes time; it should be done only when a drug is very expensive, or the discrepancy is very large, or both, or when the drug concerned is on the Dangerous Drugs List.

Controlling the overuse of drugs, which is a common problem, is usually a matter of educating health staff in the proper use of drugs.

The A/B or double-shelf system of drug stock control

The A/B or double-shelf stock control system can be used either for all drugs or only for important and life-saving drugs.

When a new drug stock is received, it should be divided into two parts that can be labelled A and B and placed separately on two shelves.

Part B should be sealed in a plastic bag or otherwise wrapped and placed on the bottom shelf. As a reminder, it should be labelled "not to be used until new order is sent".

When part A, on the top shelf, is finished, the order-form for new stock should be sent.

Part B should then be used. By the time this is finished the new stocks will have arrived.

The A/B system as described here will work only if the supply time is half the purchasing interval. If the supply time is longer, a much larger stock must be kept, and part B must be larger than part A.

Note: 'Supply time' is the time between sending an order and receiving the goods; 'purchasing interval' is the time between the arrivals of successive drug orders, usually three or six months.

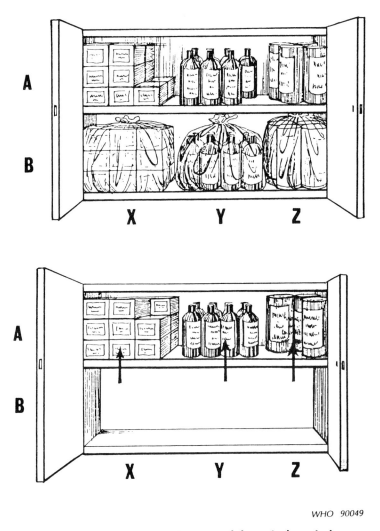

WHO 90049

The A/B or double-shelf system of drug stock control

Controlling life-saving drugs

Sometimes a patient's condition is so acute, severe or critical that only the immediate use of certain drugs can save his or her life. It is of vital importance that such drugs are always in stock; their absence in an emergency may result in a patient's death. This is an unnecessary tragedy and a failure of health-service management. To avoid this it is essential to:

— make a list of life-saving drugs
— place them together on one shelf

— check the shelf frequently or whenever drugs are issued
— order a new supply when stocks are depleted by half (using the A/B or double-shelf system described above).

Example: an emergency drug list for a rural dispensary

For severe and cerebral malaria	quinine (oral)
	quinine (injection)
Antibiotic for severe bronchopneumonia, septicaemia and acute infections	sulfamethoxazole-trimethoprim (oral)
	benzylpenicillin (injection)
Safe, all-purpose anticonvulsant	phenobarbital (oral)
For severe asthma and anaphylactic shock	epinephrine (adrenaline) injection
For severe dehydration	saline solution (intravenous)
For post-partum haemorrhage	ergometrine (injection)
Analgesic for severe injuries	pethidine (injection) *or* morphine (injection)

Note: The drugs used for emergencies and the forms in which they are used depend on local circumstances and especially on the ability of the health worker to make a clinical diagnosis and administer the drugs safely.

Prepackaging drugs for the outpatient department

A full course of treatment with tablets of a certain drug may be pre-packaged by putting it in a small envelope or folded paper before the start of a clinic or outpatient session. It is then ready when the patient needs it. This has a number of advantages:

● The patient receives the correct and full course of treatment.

● Time is saved, and waiting and queuing while tablets are counted are avoided.

● Printed instructions can be given with the packet or written on the envelope, telling the patient how and when to take the tablets. Special signs must be devised to give the same information to patients who cannot read, e.g. the sun rising on the horizon to indicate morning.

● The system is particularly useful in special clinics where standard treatments are given to all patients, e.g. iron and folic acid tablets to pregnant women.

● Observing and controlling the issue of drugs are made easier.

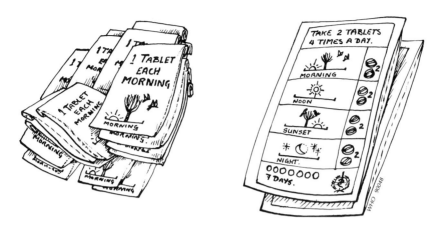

(The symbols used in these illustrations may need to be adapted for different countries).

How to prepackage drugs

The following procedure should be followed for prepackaging drugs:

1) Make a list of those drugs that are frequently prescribed.
2) Write out details of the usual treatment for each age group, e.g. 1–4 years, 5–9 years, 10–15 years, and adults.
3) Write each day's treatment in such a way that patients can easily understand it; for example:

   Adult

   Take ONE tablet three times each day:
   one on awaking
   one at midday
   one at bedtime
   and continue the treatment for . . . . . days.

4) Stencil and duplicate the instructions. If possible, use different coloured paper for each age group.
5) Obtain or make small envelopes.
6) Place the correct number of tablets for a full course of treatment in each envelope. Glue the instructions to the envelopes.

CHAPTER 3

Managing money

Learning objectives

After studying this chapter and doing Exercises 49 and 50 on pages 246–248, the health worker should be able to:

— keep accounts (i.e. make the necessary entries in a ledger)

— use a petty-cash imprest system.

Managing money in a health service is complex and responsible work, which is done mainly by accountants or finance officers. The health-worker manager of a small unit such as a health centre usually has very little responsibility for spending money. Sometimes, however, a health worker may be asked to record the spending of money (i.e. to keep accounts).

There are two types of money:

● *Invisible money, or budgetary allocation.* This is money that is not seen or handled. It is a 'paper credit' given as an allowance, allocation or warrant of funds.

For example, the government may give a health centre an allocation of $500 to draw drugs from the government medical stores. The health centre accounts for the drugs drawn from this store, with a paper called an order or requisition to be charged against the allocation. Actual money does not pass through the health centre, but a written account must be kept of each order or requisition used against the allocation (in this case $500).

● *Visible money, or cash.* This is money that is seen and handled. It is advanced to the health worker to spend for the work of the health service. It is called cash. It is not safe to have a large amount of cash at the health centre as it may be stolen. For this reason 'visible' money is usually small in amount and is called 'petty cash'.

3.1 Keeping an allocations ledger (or spending 'invisible' money)

The government (or any other organization) may allocate an amount of 'invisible' money to a health unit. It is usually for a definite purpose and can be spent only for that purpose, e.g. for drugs, equipment or transport. Accurate records of how this allocation is spent must be kept in an allocations ledger (accounts book). An allocations ledger should show the amount allocated and the detailed use of the allocation.

The layout of a typical allocations ledger is shown below.

Date	Description/Purpose	Document reference (folio no.)	Order or requisition (debit)	Allocation (credit)

Filling in an allocations ledger

The allocation of 'invisible' money may be granted either monthly, quarterly or annually. When the amount is granted, the date, the purpose and the amount are recorded in the allocations ledger. The reference number of the document that confirms the grant of the money is written in the column headed "Document reference (folio no.)", in order that the original document can be found again when necessary.

When a purchase is made, the date, the order (or requisition) and the amount are also immediately recorded. The number of the requisition form or order-form is written in the "Document reference (folio no.)" column. From this number the order (or requisition) can be found again in the files that hold copies of the order-forms or requisitions.

At certain intervals, perhaps monthly or quarterly, the amount paid out is totalled and deducted from the amount allocated (or received).

The unused balance of allocation is then 'brought forward' (B/F) and added to the new allocation for the next month, quarter or year, according to the interval chosen.

Example: An allocations ledger where a sum of $500 is granted every three months for drugs

Date	Description/Purpose	Document reference (folio no.)	Order or requisition (debit)	Allocation (credit)
1.7	Allocation for 3 months (July–Sept.)	36		500.00
3.7	Requisition	54	253.20	
15.7	Requisition	55	26.70	
1.8	Requisition	56	134.30	
5.9	Requisition	57	69.00	
	Totals		483.20	500.00
	Balance		16.80	
30.9	Balance brought forward (B/F)			16.80
1.10	Allocation for 3 months (Oct.–Dec.)	37		500.00
5.10	Requisition	58	276.80	

Note: Drugs that have been ordered will be found by referring to the file containing copies of requisitions numbers 54 to 58.

3.2 Using a petty-cash imprest system (or spending 'visible' money)

'Petty cash' means a small amount of money. Most workplaces find it convenient to have some petty cash. 'Invisible' money (allocations) can be used for large purchases such as drugs and equipment, but there are many small items that cannot be paid for with allocations, e.g. bus fares.

Petty cash is advanced to the health worker to be used exclusively for certain authorized health service needs. What the health worker is allowed to buy or pay for with petty cash may vary from one place to another. The following are some examples of the types of item that are sometimes paid for with petty cash.

Transport:	bus fares, mending bicycle punctures, petrol
Postage:	stamps, telegrams, calls from a public telephone box
Cleaning needs:	soap, detergent, antiseptic, furniture polish
Office needs:	paper, envelopes, glue, string, adhesive tape, pins
Sundries:	matches, paraffin, candles, tea, emergency supplies.

The imprest system

An imprest is an advance of cash given for a particular purpose and replenished as necessary. An imprest is always restored to its original level. In this way it is different from a grant, which is a definite amount for a definite period. An imprest may be replenished at any time when the cash balance is becoming low.

Thus, if special needs arise, the imprest cash may be spent within a week, but at other times it may last for one or two months. Whatever the period, the imprest will be replenished to the original level, provided that the money spent has been accounted for.

Suppose that a health worker is given an imprest of $40. He finds his office supplies are low, so he buys some stationery (carbon paper, stamps, glue, paper-clips) all in one week. He spends a total of $32.20, leaving an unspent balance of $7.80. He then takes his receipts and petty-cash book to his finance officer, who will give him $32.20 in cash to make the imprest up to $40 again. The imprest is now replenished. It may now take several weeks before he uses all the office supplies he bought, so that he may not need to replenish the imprest for a month or more.

An imprest is replenished only against original receipts for money spent; this prevents misuse of funds.

At any time unused cash plus disbursements must add up to the imprest level.

The petty-cash voucher

Each time money is spent from the petty-cash box, it must be recorded on a form. This form is called a petty-cash voucher. Each petty-cash voucher is numbered and is kept and filed in order.

Each petty-cash voucher must have a receipt attached to it from the person who sold the goods. If this is not possible, the voucher must be signed by the health worker in charge of the petty cash. Vouchers must be kept carefully because the finance officer, chief cashier or auditor may ask to see them at any time.

Example: A petty-cash voucher (PCV)

```
Voucher No. . . . . . . PCV 17 . . . . . . . . . . . . . . . . .

Date           . . . . . 11.12.1992 . . . . . . . . . . . . .

                    PETTY CASH VOUCHER

Goods                                      Amount
                                             $
1 packet candles                            4.25
1 box matches                               0.50
                                            4.75
Encl. receipt (to attach to the PCV)

         (by health worker who made the purchase)
Signed . . . . . . . . . . . . . . . . . . . . . . . . . . . . . . . . . . . . .

         (by finance officer)
Passed . . . . . . . . . . . . . . . . . . . . . . . . . . . . . . . .
```

Keeping petty-cash records

There are two ways of keeping petty-cash books, as described below.

The simple petty-cash book

The simple petty-cash book is used to record small amounts and where there is no need to show the breakdown of expenditure by category.

A simple petty-cash book has five columns, as shown in the following example.

Example: A simple petty-cash book

Date	Details	Voucher no.	Amount Received $	Paid out $
1.4	To imprest (original funding)	—	40.00	
2.4	Stamps	1		8.40
3.4	Bus fares	2		5.30
8.4	Telegram	3		4.20
11.4	Stamps	4		2.20
	Bicycle puncture	5		2.70
	Stationery	6		5.60
12.4	Kerosene	7		3.80
15.4	TOTAL		40.00	32.20
	Balance			7.80
16.4	Balance B/F		7.80	
	To imprest (replenishment)		32.20	

In the example above an imprest of $40 is established; seven payments have been made, totalling $32.20, using seven petty-cash vouchers, leaving a balance of $7.80. At this point the imprest is restored to the original $40 by adding the amount replenished ($32.20) to the remaining balance ($7.80).

The columnar petty-cash book

A columnar petty-cash book provides more details than the simple type. It has the advantage that each type of expenditure is recorded in a separate column. It shows not only the total spent but also how much is spent on separate items such as stamps, bus fares, office stationery, etc.

An example of a page of a columnar petty-cash book is given below. It shows the same items as the simple petty-cash example above, but in this case the amount spent is recorded in separate headed columns according to the type of expenditure. Each column is added vertically. The totals of the "Paid out (details)" columns are added horizontally. These must tally.

The original imprest level minus the total expenditure gives the balance in hand. The balance in the petty-cash book must agree with the cash held in the box.

Example: A columnar petty-cash book

Date	Details	Voucher no.	Amount		Paid out (details)			
			Received	Paid out (total)	Postage	Transport	Office	Sundry
1.4	To imprest (original funding)	1	40.00					
2.4	Stamps	2		8.40	8.40			
3.4	Bus fare	3		5.30		5.30		
8.4	Telegram	4		4.20	4.20			
11.4	Stamps	5		2.20	2.20			
	Bicycle puncture	6		2.70		2.70		
	Stationery	7		5.60			5.60	
12.4	Kerosene	8		3.80				3.80
15.4	TOTALS		40.00	32.20	14.80	8.00	5.60	3.80
	Balance			7.80				
	Balance B/F		7.80					
16.4	To imprest (replenishment)	9	32.20					

The imprest level is given in the 'Received' column. The number of each petty-cash voucher form is written in the appropriate column. In the example above, the imprest is replenished after 16 days. A larger imprest would be a serious responsibility in view of the risk of theft.

KEEP THE PETTY CASH UNDER LOCK AND KEY!

CHAPTER 4

Managing time

> ### Learning objectives
>
> **After studying this chapter and doing Exercises 51–55 on pages 248–255, health workers should be able to:**
>
> **— investigate their own and other staff members' use of time**
>
> **— plan the use of time according to the work to be carried out, i.e.**
> **arrange time-tables and schedules**
> **arrange duty rosters**
> **arrange long-term programmes**
> **annotate and use a year calendar.**

Time is not often thought of as a resource. However, it is a non-renewable resource; no event can take place unless there is time for it.

> **USING TIME EFFECTIVELY IS A MANAGEMENT SKILL**

This chapter is concerned with two aspects of the management of time:

— finding out (investigating) how staff spend time in a health service
— planing the use of time according to work to be done, using timetables, schedules, rosters and programme charts.

4.1 Finding out how staff use time

How much time is spent with patients, how much on correspondence, how much on talking to other staff, how much on visiting in the district?

These questions and others like them may be answered roughly by keeping a daily diary for a few days. An example, in the form of a table, is shown on page 196.

Health workers should make a similar table for their own activities and those of other staff members, using different headings according to their work requirements.

Example: Daily time-diary of a medical assistant in a health unit

Name of staff member . . . . Day . . . . Date . . . .

Time	Patients		People		Administration		Dis-trict	Breaks	Remarks
	OPD	Wards	Staff	Meet-ings	Office	Stock inspec-tion			
7.30	1 h								
8.30	1 h								
9.30		1 h							
10.30			10 min		20 min			30 min	Tea
11.30	1 h								
12.30			20 min		40 min				
13.30				1 h					Weekly
14.30				30 min					
Total	3 h	1 h	30 min	1 h 30 min	1 h	Nil	Nil	30 min	7 h 30 min

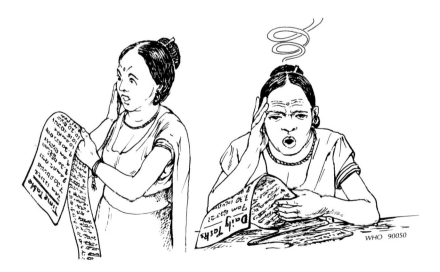

WHO 90050

Making the best use of time

Sometimes it is useful to know what proportions of time are spent on certain activities. For example, it may take four hours to travel to a distant health unit where only one hour is spent on health work, followed by four hours to return. In this case the ratio of time spent on health work to that spent in travel is 1 to 8. In such circumstances it might be decided to visit less often, and to stay overnight and work the following morning. Then the journey of four hours is followed by four hours' work on that day and four hours the next morning, and a four-hour return journey. This makes the ratio of work to travel 8 to 8, which is a more efficient use of time and gives a better service to the people.

The proportions of time spent each month on health work, travel and other activities can be shown on a diagram such as that shown in the following example:

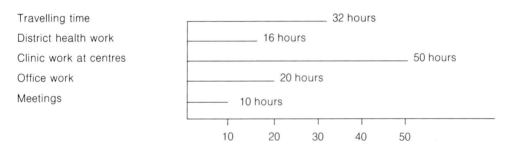

This kind of analysis will often reveal where time is being wasted or not used in the best way.

Planning time arrangements

Events are arranged in daily, weekly, monthly or yearly time periods, depending on their frequency or regularity.

Time-plans are written in various common forms known as timetables, schedules or programmes. These words are often used to mean the same thing, i.e. a time-plan. In this guide terms are used in the following way:

Timetable: for daily or weekly regularly recurring events
Schedule: for intermittent, irregular or variable events, including details of where the events take place
Roster: for duties planned for different staff members, for different times, in turn

Programme: for long-term arrangements of several different events or activities, of which the time-plan is only one part.

Time-plans in a health service

A well-managed rural health unit may need the following time-plans:

- A weekly timetable showing the time of the week when certain regular events always occur (e.g. staff meeting).
- Several schedules showing the detailed dates on which intermittent events occur and where they occur (e.g. visits to peripheral health centres or mobile clinics).
- Several duty rosters for different sections of the work (e.g. night-call, outpatient duties).
- A programme of any special health activity (e.g. a nutrition campaign).
- An annual overview of events.

Sometimes a timetable, a schedule and a roster may be combined.

4.2 Preparing a health-unit timetable

All the activities that happen regularly each week should be listed and then arranged in an appropriate timetable grid according to local working hours.

Example 1: Health centre weekly activities and timetable

List of regular activities:

Outpatients	Daily
Ward round	Three times a week
Hygiene round	Once a week
Stock inspection	Once a week
Office correspondence	Once a week
Tuberculosis/leprosy clinic	Once a week
Home visits	Twice a week
Staff meeting	Once a week
Clinical seminar	Once a week
District visit to peripheral health unit	Once a week

Time	Monday	Tuesday	Wednesday	Thursday	Friday	Saturday
7.30	Out-patients	Out-patients	Out-patients	Out-patients	Out-patients	Out-patients Ward round
10.30	BREAK					
11.00	Ward round	Office	Ward round	TB/leprosy clinic	District	Hygiene round
12.30	BREAK					
14.00	Stock inspection	Home visits	Staff meeting	Clinical seminar	Home visits	

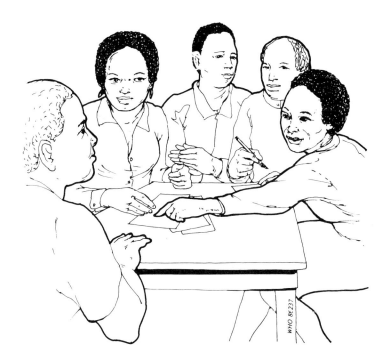

Teamwork in planning and scheduling health activities

Example 2: Community activities for one month

Month:

Day	1st week Area or district	1st week Activities	2nd week Area or district	2nd week Activities	3rd week Area or district	3rd week Activities	4th week Area or district	4th week Activities
Monday	North end of village	Home visiting	Village	Visit market on market day. Discuss hygiene	North end of village	Inform people of next day's immunization session	East end of village	Continue and complete immunization
Tuesday		Group: Health education. Nutrition demonstration	Village	Visit school. Talk with teacher. Hygiene discussion with teacher and children		Immunization session		
Wednesday		Meeting with village people. Discuss community project, e.g. digging well or latrines	East end of village	Home visiting				
Thursday	South end of village	Group health education		Group health education	South end of village	Inform people of next day's immunization session		
Friday		Health education in village school. Meeting with school teacher		General meeting with people and other community development workers		Immunization session		Write up records of immunizations. Review future equipment needs, etc.

4.3 Preparing health-unit schedules

A schedule is required when a different activity, or the same activity in a different place, occurs at intervals over time. For example, home visits may be made daily or several times a week, but they may cover different villages or different types of disease at special times. Similarly, mobile teams may travel on the same day each week but visit a different area. It may be decided to have an inspection every Monday but to inspect a different part of the health unit each week.

To make a schedule, each different activity or each different place is listed and assigned dates in turn; the whole cycle is then repeated. It is essential to have a calendar showing the dates of the chosen days in the months ahead.

Schedules for mobile team visits need a map showing routes, distances and travel times. Travel times will depend on the state of roads, the nature of the terrain (e.g. the number of hills), and other factors as well as the distance. It may be possible to leave half a team at one place while the rest go on to another, thus saving time. Returning by a circular route and visiting yet another place later in the day may also be possible.

Other factors to be considered in the schedule are the number of people in the villages or area (population density) and the days of local markets.

The following examples show schedules for mobile team visits and for supervision and maintenance checks of a health unit.

Example 1: Schedule for mobile team visits to cover eight villages

Arranged routes (see map, page 203)

Route 1:	Visit villages A, B and C. Leave half the team at A, to walk to C later. Go to B for morning clinic. Whole team at C for afternoon clinic.
Route 2:	Go to village E to catch early morning ferry. Return to D by midday to hold afternoon clinic.
Route 3:	Visit X only (long distance over mountain road).
Route 4:	Morning clinic at village Q. Short clinic at R on return.

Travel every Tuesday and Friday, thus visiting each place every two weeks.

		Villages ABC Route 1	Villages DE Route 2	Village X Route 3	Villages QR Route 4
April	Tuesday	April 04			
	Friday		April 07		
	Tuesday			April 11	
	Friday				April 14
	Tuesday	April 18			
	Friday		April 21		
	Tuesday			April 25	
	Friday				April 28
May	Tuesday	May 02			
	Friday		May 05		
	Tuesday			May 09	
	Friday				May 12
	Tuesday	May 16			
	Friday		May 19		
	Tuesday			May 23	
	Friday				May 26

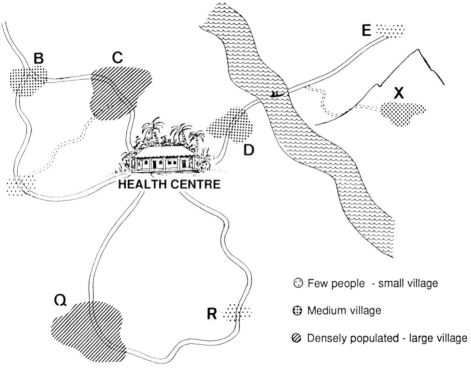

⊙ Few people - small village

⊕ Medium village

⊘ Densely populated - large village

Example 2: Schedule for supervision and maintenance checks of a health unit

To be inspected	Every Monday, as shown				
Store-room and stock ledger	April	03	Holiday	July	24
Laboratory, laboratory inventory		10	June 05		31
Building, grounds, kitchen		17	12	Aug	7
Vehicle and log-book		24	19		14
Outpatient and inpatient units	Holiday		26		21
Maternity and MCH unit	May	08	July 03	Holiday	
Office and filing systems		15	10	Sept	04
Drug stock and drug usage		22	17		11

In Example 2, each section has a special control inspection every eight weeks. This spreads the work of control and maintenance evenly over the year and takes very little time (perhaps one hour) each week.

Public holidays often occur on scheduled dates. When this happens, another time must be planned for the activity, or the inspection may wait for another eight weeks.

4.4 Preparing duty rosters

A duty roster is a time-plan for distributing work among staff members in turn.

Duty rosters are common in all types of health work. They are needed for three purposes:

— to distribute work fairly and evenly outside normal working hours (e.g. night, weekend, holiday and overtime duty)
— to distribute uninteresting or difficult work, and interesting or varied work, equally among the various members of the unit; in maternity work, for instance, midwives could rotate among the mobile team, the delivery unit and the clinic
— to divide extra duties among the whole staff; such extra duties might include supervision of the nutrition garden, making education posters, tracing defaulters and doing the hygiene inspection.

Making duty rosters fair and just to all staff members is both difficult and important. Unless they are arranged very carefully they can cause a great deal of trouble and quarrelling.

Rosters have to be changed frequently, because staff become sick, go on leave, or are transferred or promoted, or because public holidays intervene.

Two rules for duty rosters

When rotating several people (or groups) through several types of duty, there are two important rules:

- The length of time of each duty period must be the same as for all other types of duty period. A duty period may be a day or a week or a month, but all periods must be the same within a single roster.
- The number of people (or groups) working in turn must divide evenly into the number of duty stations or duty periods; for instance, three people cannot be rostered through five duty stations, or five people through three duty stations.

To make a duty roster, the date of the beginning of each new roster should be listed in the left-hand column. The duty stations should be listed across the page. Names should be filled in, in order from left to right, starting each new line one column further on.

Example: A duty roster problem

Suppose there is a group of eight nurses to work in turn through six different health centre duties, e.g. wound dressing station, injection stations, examination room, maternal and child health (MCH) clinics, delivery ward, and night duty.

According to the roster rules, the number of duty periods must be equal to, or divide evenly by, the number of people (or groups) to be rostered. In this case, there are six duty stations and eight people. Because eight does not divide evenly into six, it is not possible to make a roster.

What is the solution to this problem?

- Reduce the nurses to six groups by making two group of two nurses and four 'groups' of one nurse, or keep two nurses in reserve to be placed when others fall sick or are very busy. This permits a six-week roster.

The eight nurses are Nurses A, B, C, D, E, F, G, H.
The six nurse groups are AG, BH, C, D, E, F

Weeks beginning		Wounds	Injections	Examination room	MCH	Deliveries	Night duty
April 10	May 22	AG	BH	C	D	E	F
17	29	F	AG	BH	C	D	E
24	June 05	E	F	AG	BH	C	D
May 01	12	D	E	F	AG	BH	C
08	19	C	D	E	F	AG	BH
15	26	BH	C	D	E	F	AG

● Increase the duty periods to eight by doubling the time at two of the duty stations so that they appear twice on the roster. This permits an eight-week roster.

The eight nurses are Nurses A, B, C, D, E, F, G, H

Weeks beginning		Wounds	Injections	Exam. Room	MCH	MCH	Delivery	Delivery	Night duty
April 10	June 05	A	B	C	D	E	F	G	H
17	12	H	A	B	C	D	E	F	G
24	19	G	H	A	B	C	D	E	F
May 01	26	F	G	H	A	B	C	D	E
08	July 03	E	F	G	H	A	B	C	D
15	10	D	E	F	G	H	A	B	C
22	17	C	D	E	F	G	H	A	B
29	24	B	C	D	E	F	G	H	A

4.5 Preparing a programme chart

A programme is a plan that outlines a series of events or activities that will take place in the future. A programme usually includes *what* will be done, *where* it will take place, *who* will do it, and *when* it will occur. The time-plan is therefore only part of the total programme.

A simple programme of health education may be a series of monthly discussions in the community, when different health workers will help with discussions on various health problems. In more complex programmes, later activities depend on earlier ones; for instance, to organize a special or extra immunization programme, it may be necessary first to order the equipment (e.g. syringes). Or, if a new activity is to commence, a staff member may have to be sent on a training course, and the public must be informed.

There are several ways to make a programme chart. A convenient way is to list the activities, in the order in which they must occur, down the left side of the page, then fill in the weeks or months across the top of the page, and then show with a line opposite each planned activity the week or weeks during which it is to take place.

Example: A timed programme arrangement

To establish a new family planning clinic in health centre X

Proposed time of activities (each column represents one week)

Activities	August				September				October			
	07	14	21	28	04	11	18	25	02	09	16	23
Discuss project with health centre staff	—											
Select nurse or volunteer for training		—										
Send volunteer on two-week course					—							
Prepare material to inform the public					—							
Order equipment needed					—							
Hold meetings to inform the public							—					
Date equipment is expected										—		
First clinic												—

4.6 Preparing a year calendar

In the course of a year many things happen that are outside the normal routine. These may be matters of administration such as annual stock-taking, estimates, annual reports, and statistical returns, or they may be external events such as festivals, elections, conferences and seminars, or visits by dignitaries.

So that the whole year may be seen at once, it is very convenient to have a one-page annual calendar or year-planner pinned on the wall, with important events marked. This has two functions:

— it acts as a reminder of definite events, usually outside one's control
— it shows where it is possible to fit in new events such as special meetings or periods of travel.

Lined paper (with about 30 lines) is useful for this. Dates of the months are written down the left margin and 12×1.25 cm columns are drawn across the page, one for each month. Dates you wish to be reminded of, and dates of all public holidays, should be entered.

Example: A year calendar

Date	Jan	Feb	Mar	Apr	May	Jun	Jul	Aug	Sep	Oct	Nov	Dec
1					[PH]							
2												
3												
4												
5		x D									Elec. day	
6		x M										
7		x Q										
8									A			
9	'								N			
10				S		x M			N			
11				E		x O			U			
12				M		x H			A			
13				I					L			
14				N								
15				A					L			
16				R					E			
17									A			
18									V			
19									E			
20												
21												
22												
23												
24			[PH]									
25											[PH]	
26											[PH]	
27			[PH]									
28								[PH]				
29					[PH]							
30												
31												

Code: [hatch] Public holiday

x Visits: DMO = District Medical Officer, MOH = Ministry of Health

CHAPTER 5

Managing space

	Learning objectives

> ### Learning objectives
>
> **After studying this chapter and doing Exercises 56–59 on pages 255–259, the health-worker manager should be able to:**
> — **arrange working space in such a way that work flows smoothly and for the convenience of the patients and others who use it**
> — **show on a map the catchment area of a health service**
> — **use maps in district health work**
> — **make a sketch map of a health district.**

This chapter is concerned with two kinds of working space and how to make the best use of them in providing health care:

— the buildings or other settings where health care is given
— the geographical or 'catchment' area served by a health centre.

5.1 Arranging work-space

Good management takes care in arranging the space where staff work. Because of the small size of the building or of individual rooms, or their awkward shape, or often because no one has given the matter any thought, many health units have unsuitable space arrangements.

There are no complex rules about the arrangement of working space. Only two simple questions need to be answered:

● What work has to be done here?
● Could this space be arranged in another way that would make the work easier and suit the patients better?

Example

> A medical assistant examined adult patients at one end of a room containing a table and a chair. A nurse examined children at the other end of the room.
>
> There was no examination couch. For a full examination adults had to cross the corridor to another room. This took time, with the result that the medical assistant rarely had time to examine anybody.
>
> A good supervisor came and placed two screens beside the medical assistant's table, with a narrow bed behind them. Patients could now undress in privacy, while the medical assistant continued with the next patient. This made his work much easier, suited the patients better and avoided waiting and delays.

Note: Simple screens, consisting of a timber frame covered with cloth, are a very easy way of making extra rooms.

A common problem is lack of storage space. Stores are often much too small and become over-full, so that it is difficult to find things.

There are several possible solutions to this. One is to place lockable cupboards along a corridor. Another is to turn the office into a large store and use the store as a small office.

5.2 Arranging work-flow

One of the features of many health units is a lack of order in the way people are dealt with. In the same space there may be people sitting waiting, while others are standing in queues; people get in one another's way or impede the work of the staff. Most of these problems can be improved by attention to 'work-flow'.

Work-flow is an arrangement in which a series of work functions are coordinated in space and time so that delays are minimal. The greatest obstacle to the organization of work-flow is one of attitude. Congestion and queues are now so common in health services that most people regard them as normal or inevitable and make no effort to prevent them. Some people think that long queues show how busy and hard-working they are.

Most factories or production units provide good examples of work-flow. Whether a factory is automated or operated by human labour, procedures always follow each other in a space/time order.

In a bottling factory, for example, used bottles are received and washed, then move to the next area where they are sterilized and dried. They move to another area and are filled, then to the next stage where the caps are fixed on.

If something were to go wrong with the filling stage, for instance stocks of fruit juice were to run out, the clean and dry bottles would keep coming and pile up together in the filling room. Meanwhile the workers in the subsequent stages would have nothing to do.

This is what happens when there is a queue in a health centre: there is a delay or a blockage in one stage of a work-flow.

However, moving people like bottles in a factory is not the best way to help them. The alternatives are considered below.

Work-flow in an outpatient department

To organize work-flow in an outpatient department each stage must be examined separately. If there is a queue, it is a sign that work speed or work efficiency must be improved or that work distribution must be changed.

The usual flow in an outpatients unit is as follows:

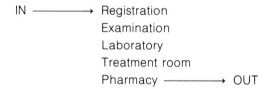

It is essential to examine the whole process. Removing a queue from one stage may result only in creating a queue at another; for instance, if registration is speeded up so that patients get their cards quickly, a queue may form outside the examination room. If the position at the examination room is improved, patients may have to wait at the pharmacy for their drugs.

EXAMINE THE WHOLE WORK-FLOW

Improving work-flow

Good work-flow has been achieved when each patient can go through each stage with only a very short waiting time. The following are some ways to avoid delays:

- Every door should be labelled so that patients know where to go.
- At registration:
  - there should be separate systems for returning and new patients;
  - returning patients should be allowed to keep their cards, or be given numbers by which their cards can be found rapidly
  - a workable filing system should be established by which record cards can be found rapidly.
- For the best use of the examination room:
  - an orderly or junior nurse should be trained to screen[1] patients in a different area, e.g. to take the history, to take the temperature, and, if there is fever, to make a blood slide;
  - patients returning daily for a course of treatment should go directly to the treatment room;
  - printed or duplicated prescriptions should be kept ready for all routine minor complaints;
  - clinic days should be established for special conditions that require more time, e.g. tuberculosis, leprosy, malnutrition;
  - appointments with busy officials should be made for less busy times.
- In the pharmacy:
  - a stock of written instructions to patients on how to take routine courses of drugs should be kept;
  - routine courses of drugs should be prepackaged (see Section 2.4).
- A *family health service* should be organized, which would be concerned with care for whole families, and with contacts between the families and the health centre staff. In such a system, a number of families from a district, a village, a number of hamlets or several streets, are assigned to a health-centre worker who is responsible for their health care. As a result, a woman need not make several visits to the health centre, say for antenatal care one day and for children's immunization another day. Instead, her own and her family's needs can be met in one visit. The

[1] In this context 'screening' means to assess everyone briefly (e.g. by interview and a quick examination) to ensure that those who do not need to see the doctor or another senior health worker are dealt with by other members of the staff instead. The doctor can then give sufficient time and attention to the patients who need a level of medical care that a medical assistant alone cannot give.

health worker receives and examines the family and advises or prescribes for them at one time, and then sees them at home in the course of visits to the community. For convenience, or because each health worker cannot have a separate treatment area, it is usually necessary to maintain a clinical area for dressings, injections, fitting of contraceptives, etc. to which people are referred, returning to their own health worker before leaving the health centre.

Such a family health service has several advantages:

— Unnecessary journeys are avoided, especially for mothers with several children. Families visit the centre less often, apart from special visits for treatment for a particular member (e.g. to collect drugs for leprosy or tuberculosis). Women attending antenatal clinics can bring their children at the same time.
— Staff have much more job satisfaction. The varied activities and sense of responsibility stimulate interest. Families feel they have a friend at the health centre.
— The family is seen as a total unit, and a health problem can be seen in its entirety. The history obtained is the family history; the same information is not requested several times.
— Less skilled health workers are better able to screen patients so that only those with problems that need more skilled medical or nursing care take up the time and effort of a supervising nurse or doctor. Usually most people can be cared for by the less skilled health workers, and only the more serious problems have to be referred to the more highly qualified staff.
— Work is more efficient because time and other resources are used better. Training programmes can be set up to enable health workers to deal with their expanded role as family health workers. Staff can be rotated in 'family duty' so that those working in the treatment area may become family health workers for a time.

5.3 Defining the catchment area

'Catchment area' is a term borrowed from geography, where it means that part of a land surface from which rain water is collected and flows into a river or lake.

When the term is applied to a health unit, it means the area from which patients come to the health service. In the case of a regional or district hospital the catchment area is the whole region or district; for a health centre it would be the villages around the health centre, and for a small treatment post or aid-post it might be only one village.

When there are several health centres in a district their catchment areas may overlap, as shown in the following diagram.

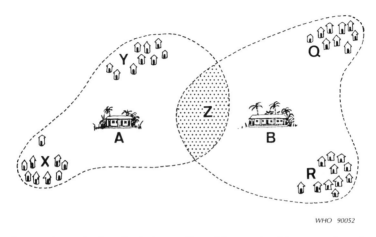

WHO 90052

People living in the shaded area Z could go to health centre A or B

People in villages X and Y go to health centre A, and people in Q and R go to B.

> **IDENTIFY THE CATCHMENT AREA**

The idea of the catchment area is most important because it defines the area of responsibility of a health unit. A health unit is meant to give a complete health service to all the people and communities in its catchment area. This means that all matters affecting health within the catchment area are management responsibilities of the health unit. To know what these responsibilities are, the catchment area must be defined.

5.4 Using maps in district health work

A district health centre without maps is like a physician without a clinical record: it is missing an important guideline. The following are some of the many uses of maps in health work:

- To show distances to various health units and villages. Distance can be measured in kilometres or in travelling-time. Travelling-time is the more important for health work.

  With the aid of a map that shows bad roads, winding roads, mountains or ferries, the travelling-time to each place should be calculated and listed.

- To plan routes. In district health work it may be convenient and time-saving to visit two or three places on the same day. Suitable routes can be planned with the help of a map.

- To decide on travelling methods. Some routes may be covered by regular bus services; these can be marked on the map. Other roads may be impassable except by jeep, or impassable during certain seasons.

- To learn the population distribution and density of an area. The main centres of population are shown on the map. The density of population (number of people per square kilometre) can also be shown. This helps in deciding how long a clinic session or health campaign is likely to take.

- To learn of the different types of community in an area. There may be villages of different types — for instance, the standardized housing of plantation workers, or semi-urban communities in large villages, or very scattered farms.

- To obtain information about the community environment. Maps can give a great deal of information about the environmental features that influence health; for instance, a map can show all the main water sources such as rivers, wells and springs and whether they are dammed or piped. A detailed map could also show the number and distribution of sanitary facilities in an area.

- To show the topography of an area, i.e. its physical features — mountains, rivers and vegetation, and whether the vegetation is forest, bush or cultivated land.

- To show public buildings, particularly those that can be used for health work such as clinics or meetings. Schools, community halls, administration offices or large warehouses may be borrowed when necessary for different types of health work.

- Information obtained from health surveys is sometimes shown on maps by means of coloured pins; for example, one pin for every 10 or 20 patients with a certain disease, such as leprosy, may be stuck in the part of the map that shows where these patients live. The distribution of pins will then indicate the distribution of leprosy in the area. This, in turn, will show the most convenient places for mobile clinics.

Not all features can be recorded on one map. Usually several are needed, each giving a different kind of information.

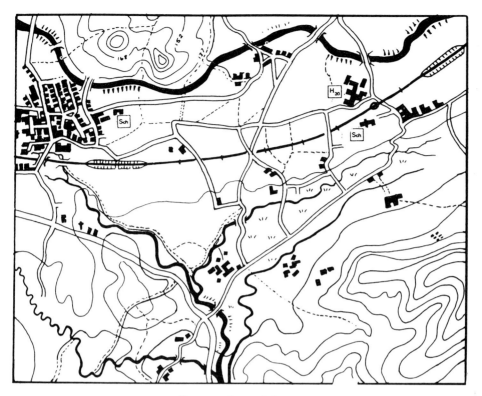

Topography and rivers

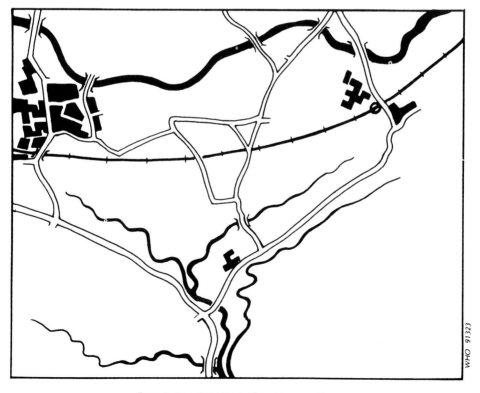

Population density and water supplies

WHO 91323

On the previous page are two maps of the same place, one showing topography and rivers, and the other showing population density and water supplies. Many of the symbols used on maps are identified in Section 5.5.

5.5 Making a health-district sketch map

Geographical mapping is difficult and time-consuming. Each feature must be in exact proportion. A health worker does not have the skill or the time to make accurate, in-scale, geographical maps.

Maps may often be obtained from the local government office or land department. They may be unnecessarily detailed, but the main features needed for health work may be traced from the map on transparent paper and then transferred to a large card and hung on a wall. If there is no official map, a rough sketch-map of the whole area is better than none.

A code of signs should be prepared to use on the map, for the features that must be shown, such as those indicated with the examples below.

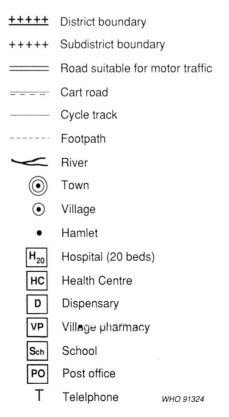

＋＋＋＋＋	District boundary
＋＋＋＋＋	Subdistrict boundary
══════	Road suitable for motor traffic
＝ ＝ ＝ ＝	Cart road
────────	Cycle track
- - - - - - -	Footpath
∽	River
⊙	Town
⊙	Village
•	Hamlet
H₂₀	Hospital (20 beds)
HC	Health Centre
D	Dispensary
VP	Village pharmacy
Sch	School
PO	Post office
T	Telelphone

WHO 91324

CHAPTER 6

Managing paperwork

Learning objectives

After studying this chapter the health worker should be able to:

— **organize an office in a health unit**

— **write referral and other official letters**

— **set up a filing system**

— **arrange and index a health-unit office system.**

Paperwork, mainly correspondence and the maintenance and use of records, is an essential part of the management of a health service, and almost all health activities involve paperwork. Its quality and efficiency play a large part in the effectiveness of health care activities and programmes. Without a well ordered records system, for example, neither clinical care nor community health work can be monitored or controlled. Paperwork is the communication system (correspondence), the information system (reports) and the memory system (records, registers) of a health service. This chapter deals with the writing of referral and other official letters, and with the organization of a records system.

6.1 The functions of an office in a health centre

An office is a place where paperwork is done and documents and letters are stored. It is not always a whole room: it may be simply a table or a desk or a corner of a room.

Some examples of the paperwork essential to the main functions of a health unit are shown on the next page.

Activity or function	Paperwork
Correspondence (letter-writing)	
Patient problems	Patient-referral letters
Administrative problems	Letters to and from supervisors
Health care activities	
Patient attendance	Registration
Examination and diagnosis	Clinical records
Treatment	Laboratory register
Inpatient admission	Ward register
Discharge	Discharge letter/form
Special diseases	Tuberculosis/leprosy registers
Maternal care	Antenatal cards
Child care	Child health cards
Environmental survey	Report forms
General activity	Monthly report forms
Health education	Posters, leaflets
Staff management	
Staff problems	Staff files
Administration of funds and equipment	
Ordering	Requisition (order) forms
Storing	Stock ledgers
Issuing	Issue vouchers and inventories
Funds	Cash books, receipts and petty-cash vouchers
Staff meetings	Minutes of meetings

In some countries a family file combines several of the papers listed under "Correspondence" and "Health care activities". Sometimes a health centre keeps records of the births and deaths that occur in its catchment area.

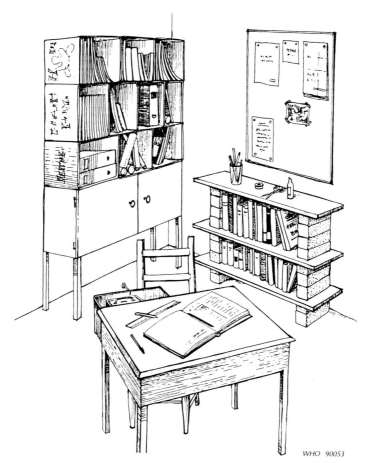

Note: Bookcase made of bricks and planks of wood
       Cupboard made of packing cases
       Notice-board made of three-ply wood.

Practical office arrangement

6.2 How to write official letters

There is an internationally accepted way of stating facts in official correspondence. However, the exact place on a page where these facts are written varies from country to country.

One correspondence format is shown below and followed by an example of a letter written in this format.

Address (coming from)

Date/Month/Year
Reference no.

Name (to whom letter is written)
Address

Reference

Dear Sir/Madam/or title and surname,

Subject underlined

    With reference to your letter dated . . . , reference no. . . . ,
. . . .

Final greeting (e.g. Yours faithfully)

Signature

Title and name, or name and qualification.
(Typed or clearly written in capitals).

Example: An official letter

The World's Best Health Centre
Village Super
DISTRICT XYZ

4th September 1992

Our ref. 56

Dr Noit
District Medical Officer
P.O. Box 493
DISTRICT XYZ

Your ref. HC/VS/879

Dear Dr Noit,

Visit to the W.B. Health Centre

With reference to your letter dated 10th August 1992, we are glad to hear that you will visit us towards the end of this month.

In answer to your question, I am pleased to tell you there is a guest-house, and we have reserved accommodation for you there.

Attached to this letter is a list of drugs and some few items which are in very short supply. If you could bring these with you, it would help us.

Yours sincerely,

ABDULLAH MOHAMMED
(Senior M.O. in charge)

MAKE CARBON COPIES OF ALL OFFICIAL LETTERS

How to write a letter referring a patient

When a patient is referred to a health centre at a higher level for further advice and treatment, a letter containing accurate details should be sent. This information will help the medical officer who sees the patient to understand the history and background of the patient's condition and treatment to date.

The following rules are a guide to referral letter-writing.

- Use the customary format for official letters.
- In place of the subject heading, write the patient's name and age.
- State the actual date when the patient was first examined (do not use statements such as 'one week ago', which may lead to confusion if there is a delay in referral).
- State the approximate date (week or month) when the patient first became ill.
- Give a summary of the main complaint, history and clinical findings.
- Give the results of any laboratory investigations.
- Most important, give full details of all treatment to date, including doses of drugs.
- Include a polite request for advice and treatment.
- Sign the letter with your name and write your official title (e.g. medical assistant or nurse-in-charge) as the person referring the patient.
- Write the patient's address, and the name and address of the patient's nearest relative, at the bottom of the letter.

Example: A referral letter

Maternity Clinic
World's Best Health Centre
Village Super
DISTRICT XYZ

11th September 1992

The Obstetrics Consultant
District Hospital
DISTRICT XYZ

Dear Doctor,

Mrs Latuma Ally, age 30 years (approx.)

I saw the above-named, who carries this letter, for the first time today. It was her first visit to the health centre, although she is about 36 weeks pregnant (she does not remember her last menstrual period).

She complains of swelling of the feet for the past 2 weeks (since the end of August). She has no other complaint.

On examination I found albumin in the urine and the blood pressure was 140/100 mmHg.

She seems to have pre-eclamptic toxaemia and therefore needs hospital admission.

I have sedated her with tab. phenobarbital 50 mg for the journey.

We send her, kindly requesting your further advice and treatment.

Thank you.

Yours sincerely,

Mrs Ainal Lunani
(Nurse-midwife)

Patient's address:	Relative (brother):
Grocer shop	Halfani Ally
Green Village	Shoemaker
District XYZ	Green Village
	District XYZ

6.3 Setting up a filing system

As stated before, an office is concerned with the organization of paper-work. An office receives, stores and transmits pieces of paper of all types, including letters, receipts, invoices, reports, patients' record cards, minutes of meetings, pamphlets, leaflets, and drug advertisements.

Sometimes documents are piled on desks so that it is difficult to find anything. Important documents are often placed in unknown files and are therefore lost. To make sure that any paper can be found whenever it is needed, a filing system must be set up.

A filing system is an arrangement by which different types of papers are placed in separate files so that they can be found again rapidly. A good filing system should have the following qualities:

● There must be a place for every type of paper normally found in the health unit (an *inclusive* system).
● It must be simple, so that staff members can maintain it (a *simple* system).
● It must be possible to find papers rapidly when needed (*retrievability*).

Filing arrangements (filing categories)

There are several methods of filing used throughout the world. These are:

— alphabetical
— numerical
— by subject
— geographical

These methods can be used in health units in the ways described below. Often two or more systems may be used together.

Alphabetical filing

The files are arranged in alphabetical order, according to the first letters of the main name of the staff member or patient. This system is used when there are large numbers of papers on similar subjects. In health services it is the most useful for staff files.

Each staff member has an individual file. In it are recorded personal particulars, employment and salary details, leave dates, increment dates, and any correspondence relating to personal problems.

Numerical filing

Each person is given a number and the files or record cards are then filed accordingly. However, a cross-reference file is needed in case, for example, patients lose their number cards.

Filing by subject

Filing by subject is the most useful system for general purposes in small health units.

All papers, documents, letters, etc. that do not belong to any existing file should be listed. A file should then be established for each subject category.

An example of such a list follows:

Correspondence
Correspondence about patients (copies of referral letters)

Correspondence with supervisor or administrator (e.g. district or regional office at a higher level than the health unit)

All other correspondence (staff correspondence, in staff members' files)

Funds and finance
Requisition forms
Receipts
Issue vouchers
Petty-cash vouchers
Inventories

Geographical filing

There should be a file for each village, containing information such as names of leaders, dates of markets, special problems, travelling times and distances, bus services, etc. This is particularly useful for supervising district work, such as mobile clinics or home visiting.

Arranging and indexing a filing system

Filing does not always achieve its main objective, which is *to allow any paper to be found any time it is needed*, because papers are often placed in the wrong file, or files are not arranged in any order, or files are not *indexed*.

An index is a list (usually alphabetical) that refers to the place where an item or article may be found. For example, a book has an index at the back, which refers to a page in the text where a particular subject is found.

A filing index refers to the name or number of the file or register where certain topics are recorded. Such a list can be typed and placed on a wall-board in an office. An example of a health-unit office index is shown below:

Information	*Location*
Administrative and other letters	Files, top shelf
Cash book	Right-hand drawer of desk
Clinical records	Box in outpatient department
Discharge forms	Ward table
Inventories	Store cupboard
Issue vouchers	Store cupboard
Leprosy cards	Box in outpatient department
Monthly reports	File, second shelf
Petty-cash vouchers	Right-hand drawer of desk
Receipts	Store cupboard
Requisition forms	Store cupboard
Stock ledger	Store cupboard
Tuberculosis cards	Box in outpatient department
Village information	By name, third shelf

Registers or ledgers

Not all records in a health unit consist of loose papers. A number of items are recorded in large books usually called registers or ledgers.

Where to find files, registers and ledgers

Files, registers and ledgers are best kept where they are used; for example, the laboratory register is kept in the laboratory, the admissions register in the ward, the stock ledger and receipts file in the storeroom or cupboard, correspondence in the office, and patients' files in the outpatient department. Wherever they are kept, they need a definite place on a shelf or in a cupboard where they can be found easily.

Where a number of files are kept in an office the shelves should be clearly labelled. The place where each document is kept is recorded in the office index.

Office accessories

In addition to documents there are office accessories, for which space must be provided on a shelf or in a cupboard. These accessories include stationery and envelopes, official forms, glue, scissors, adhesive tape, wrapping paper and string, pens, pencils and ink, stencils and duplicators.

Exercises

Exercise 37 (III.1) Inventory of equipment

Objective: To be able to draw up and check an inventory of equipment.

Individual work

Draw up a list of all the equipment you can see in the room in which you work. Mark each item "E" if you think it is expendable and "NE" if not expendable. Note the quantity of each item, and, where applicable, its state of repair (serviceable/unserviceable/serviceable after repair). Compare your list with the room inventory, if available.

Group work

Consolidate individual lists, grouping all non-expendable items together for each room, and all expendable items separately. (Discuss the exact nature of particular items when in doubt.) Compare the consolidated list with the previously available inventory, and enter for each item:

s — *s*erviceable (in a good state of repair)
r — needing *r*epair
u — *u*nserviceable (beyond repair)
m — *m*issing (i.e. on the room inventory, but not listed by health worker).

Discuss where to keep records of expendable and non-expendable items, and what should be done about unserviceable and missing items. Discuss who is in charge of the equipment inventory, and if necessary assign responsibility for it.

Exercise 38 (III.1) Requisition of supplies

Objective: To be able to requisition (order or re-order) expendable equipment to meet requirements within a budgetary allocation.

Individual work

Review the list of equipment prepared in Exercise 37 and estimate your monthly requirements for the expendable items on the list, given your usual work-load. If a suitable catalogue is available, fill in a specimen monthly requisition form.

Group work

Consolidate individual requisitions, item by item, and calculate the total value of the monthly requisition of expendable supplies. Determine whether the value of the requisition and supplies falls within the monthly budgetary allocation for equipment and supplies (the amount to be specified by the medical officer or medical assistant — or some arbitrary estimate made). If *not*, review the requirements specified by each health worker for the *most costly* items so as to reduce excessive demands, if this is indicated. Discuss what is desirable and what is feasible. Revise the requisition item by item until its total value falls within the stated amount.

Discuss how such a requisitioning process can best be undertaken routinely in the health unit, to whom the requisition must be addressed, how the amount available for equipment and supplies (budgetary allocation) is calculated, the availability of different catalogues for comparison of specifications and prices, etc. Discuss how this procedure would apply in the case of non-expendable equipment.

Exercise 39 (III.1) Storage of expendables

Objective: To be able to store expendable supplies in an orderly way.

Individual work

Make a drawing of a storage cabinet to hold stocks of the following items:

5 kg cleaning clothes
3 kg gauze
5 kg cotton
6 kg soap
20 litres methanol
2 litres ethanol
2000 disposable syringes (2 ml)
2000 hypodermic needles (reusable)
1000 wooden tongue-depressors
2000 swabsticks
1000 test-tubes (disposable)
10 1-litre glass jars with lids
0.5 kg stains (laboratory)
5 kg detergent

20 rolls adhesive tape
3 litres disinfectant liquid
5 metal boxes $20 \times 30 \times 5$ cm
5000 record cards
200 writing paper pads
1000 envelopes
50 pencils
20 ballpoint pens
10 erasers

(*Hint*: some grouping of items (e.g. office supplies, liquids, glassware) might be helpful for storage purposes and for recording in a ledger.)

After grouping the items in a few categories, indicate a code, e.g. A, B, C, etc., for each category and show on your drawing where you would store each item. For this purpose, mark each storage compartment (shelf/rack/drawer) with a subdivision of the code (A1, A2 . . . Z9) and write the appropriate code after each supply item (e.g. soap C5, record cards D1).

Group work

Review the list of expendable supplies and discuss the groupings that have been suggested. Adopt an acceptable common grouping for further steps.

Review the health workers' design of storage compartments and the suggested arrangements for storing supplies.

Select a design, and agree on a suitable storage cabinet. Using the first three columns of the sample page of a stock ledger (see page 166), code the shelves/racks/drawers and rewrite the list of supplies in alphabetical order within each group, showing item reference number, item designation, and location code in storage.

Go to the storeroom, observe the existing lay-out, and discuss how to make use of the results of this exercise.

Exercise 40 (III.1) Keeping a stock ledger

Objective: To be able to maintain a stock ledger.

Individual work

Use the format of a stock ledger (such as that shown on page 166) and record the amounts of each item listed in Exercise 39 under "stock in hand on 1.4.93". Use one page for each group of equipment and supplies. From the stock, assume that an issue of the following items is made on 14.4.93 to each of the four district midwives:

Supplied to one midwife

Soap	0.6 kg
Cotton	0.5 kg
Gauze	1 kg
Methanol	1 litre
Disinfectant	0.5 litre
Record cards	200
Syringes 2 ml	50
Needles for the syringes	50

Record these issues on the pages of the ledger.

Assume that an order received on 20.4.93 from the government medical stores contains the following items:

Syringes (2 ml, reusable)	100
Disinfectant	2 litres
Soap	4 kg
Test-tubes (disposable)	200

Enter these under the appropriate headings in the ledger and compute the stock in hand on 1.5.93, assuming no other supply movements meantime.

Group work

Compare the results obtained for stock in hand on 1.5.93, and review the way in which each health worker has made the various entries. After discussion, agree on the 'proper' way of recording and on 'correct' figures for stock in hand.

Then discuss the assignment of responsibility for maintaining stock ledgers, review the functioning of the existing procedures, and decide whether any of the steps practised in this exercise need to be introduced in your routine work.

Exercise 41 (III.1) Maintenance and repair

Objective: To be able to take appropriate action in case of equipment needing maintenance or repair.

Individual work

Refer to Exercise 37, in which the state of repair of the non-expendable equipment (serviceable, unserviceable, serviceable after repair) was noted.

Take a closer look at each item of the listed equipment in your working place. Observe its state of cleanliness, and the orderly arrangement of that equipment. Note the items that need some action and write down what you suggest should be done (e.g. dusting, washing, repainting, polishing, disinfecting, tightening) or the exact nature of the needed repair. Then ask yourself *who* should ask for, and who would undertake, the suggested maintenance or repair: write this down. Decide who has the necessary *authority* to get this done (this will vary with the nature of the work, who will do it, and the cost of doing it).

Group work

Review the list of items in need of maintenance or repair, and the different types of maintenance or repair tasks, and agree on a common list.

Then review *who* is assigned responsibility for requesting, and for carrying out, the maintenance or repair work. If this is not clear, assign each type of task specifically to a particular person (member of staff). For each type of task, review who has authority to get the job done.

Discuss the functioning of the current system of maintenance and repair on the basis of the observed needs, and note what might be introduced into the system, if necessary, to ensure its effectiveness in keeping the equipment in a good state of maintenance and repair.

Discuss any updating needed in staff job descriptions to apply the results of this exercise.

Special group work

Objectives: To assess the functioning of a health care unit and to suggest means of improving the work-flow.

Review the results of Exercises 37 to 41. List the points that need attention in order to improve the work-flow.

If the group considers that the work-flow can be improved, subgroups should be given the following tasks:

Equipment changes. List what could be done:

— to order missing equipment
— to repair damaged equipment
— to rearrange equipment so that it is readily available
— to put the work area in good order
— to maintain the functioning and arrangement of the equipment so that the work may continue smoothly.

Changes in work performance. List your suggestions in relation to:

— additional staff that may be needed
— whether volunteers can be trained for some tasks
— whether the staff should have further training to improve their performance
— how improvements in work performance could be maintained.

Changes in work arrangements. Describe any changes that could be made in work arrangements for the unit, such as:

— assigning specific days for certain kinds of patients (e.g. Wednesdays for tuberculosis patients)
— packaging drugs or supplies
— preparing stocks of duplicated written instructions to patients to avoid rewriting
— conducting discussion groups to make teaching of patients more effective and efficient
— health education of patients in groups.

Discuss the subgroups' suggestions. Determine which are feasible in the health centre. List these for consideration.

Exercise 42 (III.2) Adapting a standard drug list to local conditions

Objective: To be able to select drugs that suit the specific needs of the population of a given area.

Individual work

Read Chapter 2, Section 2.2. Review the example on pages 177–178. Set criteria for selecting drugs that a village health worker might dispense. According to these criteria, list the drugs that you think could be entrusted to a village health worker. Then study the following situation:

A one-day clinic is held once a week in a remote area with a small town and several surrounding villages. Its main function is maternal and child care, but the staff from the health centre should be prepared to treat minor ailments, injuries, and emergencies. The population of the area is about 5500; this includes 2400 adults (more than 18 years old), of whom 875 are women of childbearing age, and 560 children under 5 years, of whom 120 are under 1 year.

Maternal care	Child care	Minor ailments and injuries
Activities	*Activities*	*Activities*
antenatal care	nutrition education	Treatment for:
family planning	immunization	wounds and fractures
		bites
		belly pains
		headache
		fever
Drug list	*Drug list*	*Drug list*
iron sulfate	Vaccines	acetylsalicylic acid
tetanus toxoid	polio	gentian violet
sulfadimidine	measles	penicillin
vitamins	DPT	phenobarbital
Other materials	BCG	benzyl benzoate
contraceptives		auroomycin ointment
protein		oral rehydration salts
supplements		piperazine
		mepacrine

Calculate the quantities of these drugs you should take to meet the needs of the village population for the one-day clinic. Show clearly how many people you expect in each of the above categories, and the quantities of drugs you expect that they will need.

Group work

Compare the sets of criteria proposed by the individual health workers, discuss them, and agree on a short-list of the more useful criteria.

Review the lists of drugs selected by individual health workers, and agree on a common list that satisfies the criteria agreed by the group.

Then review the requirements estimated by individual health workers for the one-day clinic. First, discuss the expected numbers of clients of various types; second, discuss the average number of doses to be issued to each; and third, work out the quantity of each drug that should be taken along.

Exercise 43 (III.2) Stocking drugs

Objective: To be able to stock drugs so as to ensure their availability, accessibility and safety.

Individual work

Review the list of standard drugs available to the health centre. List the life-saving drugs as one group; divide all the other common drugs into eight to twelve groups according to their uses, e.g. 'analgesic and anti-pyretic', 'cardiovascular', 'dangerous'. Write down which drugs fall into each group.

Applying the 'A/B' shelf system illustrated on page 185, design a storage cabinet that will satisfy four criteria:

— give easy access to life-saving drugs
— show at a glance when stocks of common drugs become critically low
— keep a month's reserve of each group always in stock
— keep the dangerous drugs in safe custody.

Record where each group of drugs would be found.

Group work

Review the proposed groups of drugs and compare them with those in use in the health centre; discuss the advantages and disadvantages of various systems, and select the system that seems most practical. Check the lists of drugs in each group, discussing and resolving possible differences between the lists made by individual health workers. Review the suitability of the proposed storage cabinet designs for the selected drug groups, and choose a practical design that satisfies the four criteria above. Agree on a coding for racks, bins or drawers.

Then go to the drug store of the health centre and discuss what aspects, if any, of the system produced in this exercise might be usefully introduced. Bring this to the attention of the head of the centre.

Exercise 44 (III.2) Monitoring a drug stock-card system

Objective: To be able to keep up to date a record of the stock and flow of drugs.

Individual work

Choose one group of drugs from among those agreed upon in Exercise 43. Record each drug in the group on a card like that shown on page 182. (You will need to prepare some 'dummy' cards.)

Obtain from the drugs store-keeper the original records of the drugs in the chosen group.

For each drug in the group, *copy* onto your set of cards from the original record:

— the stock in hand just before the last consignment but one was received by the general medical stores (GMS)
— the amount received in the consignment before last from GMS
— the amount issued to the various users at specified dates between the consignment before last and the last consignment from GMS
— the amount received in the last consignment from GMS
— the expiry dates of the supplied batches of drugs.

Then compare the stock in hand after each receipt and issue. After recording this information, file cards together in alphabetical order.

Group work

Review the entries made by each health worker, and verify the correctness of the calculations. Discuss what purposes such a stock-card system serves, what additional information could be put on the cards to make the system fully reliable and practical, and how the operation of the system may be supervised.

Discuss what should be done when the above exercise cannot be undertaken because the original records do not contain the necessary information. Record your ideas and bring them to the attention of the store-keeper.

Exercise 45 (III.2) Monitoring drug use

Objective: To be able to assess whether the available amounts of drugs are used efficiently.

Individual work

Select the same group of drugs as in Exercise 44, and review the information on the 'dummy' stock cards for that group, with a view to finding out the following:

— whether any drug was out of stock at some point between the consignment before last and the last consignment (if so, note down which, and when it was out of stock)
— what amounts of each drug have been consumed between the last two consignments (write down the amounts)
— the mean *monthly* consumption of each drug (record this against each drug, including any that ran out of stock)
— what proportion of the latest 'stock in hand' has been consumed in the interval between the two consignments (record for instance 200/300 or 2/3 or 66%, noting that in some cases the proportion may be more than 100%, for instance 150%).

Group work

Review the statements as follows:

1) Prepare a consolidated list of drugs that ran out of stock. For each drug, review the monthly consumption, and calculate how many courses of

treatment (patients) it represents. Estimate how many patients were probably denied subsequent treatment because of drug shortage. Given the date at which these drugs ran out, calculate what amount should be requisitioned to avoid running short. Were appropriate amounts requisitioned? Were the requisitioned amounts supplied? Were they outdated, damaged, or discarded for any other reason? Determine what quantity of these 'fast-moving' drugs should be kept on shelf 'A' and how much on shelf 'B' to anticipate future shortages.

2) From the list of drugs that remained available until the later consignment, note the five to ten least consumed drugs in proportion to the latest stock in hand (for instance, below 33%). Check whether the amounts of the last two consignments were the amounts requisitioned.

Exercise 46 (III.2) Preparing a drug requisition

Objective: To be able to prepare drug requisitions to meet requirements.

Individual work

Review one by one each drug on the 'dummy' stock cards you prepared in Exercise 44. Check in each case whether the drug is *brand-name* (BN), and if so whether there is a recommended, WHO-certified, cheaper, *generic drug* (GD). Whenever there is such an alternative, make a note of it on the dummy stock card.

Sort out the cards for the 'fast-moving' drugs (i.e. those that run out of stock). For each such drug, refer to a price list and calculate the quantity of generic drug that could have been obtained for the price of the previous consignment of brand-name equivalent. Note these amounts (e.g. 300 doses BN cost as much as 1000 doses GD). Then, applying the recorded average consumption per patient, calculate whether ordering the reliable generic alternatives would be likely to cover requirements over the entire period between two consignments. If you find that it would, you should requisition these amounts of generic drugs instead of the insufficient quantities of brand-name drugs ordered previously. If you find that it would not, you must make a further analysis.

Find out which are the 'slow-moving' drugs (as determined in Exercise 45). Check their expiry dates and estimate from the recorded average monthly consumption how long the requirements are likely to be met by the available stock. If you do not need to requisition these drugs you can use the money you would have spent on them to obtain more of the fast-moving drugs instead. Calculate the quantities of fast-moving drugs you could obtain for the money saved by not re-ordering the slow-moving drugs.

Finally, review the remaining drugs, to find out in which cases demand exceeded the amount supplied in the consignment before last. In each such case determine whether you can replace a brand-name drug by a reliable generic drug, and, if you can, increase the amount of the drug you requisition so that you may meet requirements without adding to the cost.

Exercise 47 (III.2) Analysing drug prescriptions

Objective: To be able to examine factors that contribute to high use of drugs in the health centre.

Individual work

Collect and review the prescriptions that patients presented to the dispenser or pharmacist on one day (or up to a total of 30 prescriptions). Summarize them as follows:

Prescription no.	Drug name and type[1]	BN/GD	Unit (pills or vials)	Amount prescribed

1) Count the total number of different drugs prescribed on that day.
2) Count the number of prescriptions with one, two, three, four, five, or six or more drugs. Which is the most commonly prescribed number of drugs?
3) Count the number of prescriptions containing drugs of each type[1]. Which drug type is most prescribed?
4) Count the number of prescribed brand-name drugs; calculate what proportion of the total number of drugs prescribed are brand-name drugs, and how many of the prescribed brand-name drugs have a reliable generic equivalent.

---

[1] Refer to the list of essential drugs on pages 177 and 178.

5) List the *three most frequently* prescribed drugs and record for each:

— the minimum amount prescribed
— the maximum amount prescribed
— the mean amount prescribed.

Group work

Review the findings, and discuss the frequencies of prescriptions containing one, two and three different drugs, and the significance of the observed frequencies. Discuss:

— the group of drugs most frequently prescribed in relation to the needs of patients
— the proportion of brand-name drugs prescribed
— the availability of reliable generic equivalents in relation to experienced drug shortages.

Discuss the amounts prescribed of the three most frequently issued drugs in relation to the efficacy of treatment, and in all cases seek the medical prescriber's explanation for their frequent use.

Exercise 48 (III.2) Assessing patients' use of drugs

Objective: To be able to assess and influence the degree to which patients comply with prescribed treatment.

Individual work

Collect prescriptions from ten consecutive patients and arrange to interview each of them before you issue the prescribed drugs. Prepare a set of written questions to ascertain whether the patient:

1) has heard about the prescribed treatment, and from where
2) trusts the treatment for efficacy
3) fears side-effects of the treatment (if so, what)
4) would have preferred some other kind of treatment (if so, what)
5) intends to take the full course of prescribed treatment
6) knows how to take the prescribed treatment (number of drugs, number of pills, number of times each drug should be taken each day and for how many days).

Record each patient's answers on a separate sheet of paper with the patient's name and your own initials, and attach a copy of the prescription. After the interview, correct the patient's misunderstandings, relieve fears, and explain in detail how to take the prescribed treatment. Ask the patient to see you again at the next control visit, and to *bring back any unused medicines*.

On control (or home) visit, find out (and record) whether:

7) the condition has improved (not at all, little, much, very much)
8) the patient has taken the full course of treatment (if not, collect any unused medicine)
9) the patient wishes to continue the treatment or to have different treatment.

Group work

After all the answers have been collected, analyse the findings of the study in the following order:

— results of treatment (unknown/not improved/little improved/much improved/very much improved)
— compliance with prescribed treatment (unknown/treatment completed/treatment not completed)
— attitude towards treatment (unknown/does not want to continue this treatment/does not want any other treatment/wants to continue this treatment/wants other treatment).

Exercise 49 (III.3) Maintaining accounts I (allocation ledger)

Objective: To be able to maintain accounts on an allocation ledger.

Individual work

Draw up a list of equipment, supplies and services provided to the health centre for which no staff member makes a direct (cash) payment. Find out (from official correspondence, government rules and other documentation available in the health centre) what allocations of credit ('invisible money') are available to the officer-in-charge for procuring the listed equipment, supplies and services. An allocation will have a specific *name* and will specify the amount of *money* that may be spent over a stated period of *time*, e.g. "Allocation for maintenance and repairs: $100 a year".

Show in a table what kinds of equipment and supplies and services can be obtained against each allocation. Then outline a dummy allocation ledger, containing all information required by the administration for granting or renewing an allocation of credit.

Group work

Review the lists of equipment and supplies provided against various allocations, and record the names of allocations available to the health centre and the corresponding amounts and time periods. Review the information suggested as being required in an allocation ledger and agree on an appropriate outline for a ledger. Finally, discuss what authority grants an allocation, who is authorized to requisition equipment and supplies, who is responsible for seeing that a proposed expenditure can be accommodated within the credit available, and who is responsible for submitting periodic statements of balance-of-account to the granting authority.

Review the current functioning of this system in the health centre, and note which of the points discussed here might improve the system. Discuss the role of cost estimates, sealed bids, and certified bills in managing allocation money.

Exercise 50 (III.3) Maintaining accounts II (petty-cash book)

Objective: To be able to keep correct accounts of imprest and expenditure.

Individual work

List items of supply or sundries used in the health centre which are paid for directly by members of the health team. Then list members of the health team who maintain a petty-cash account to meet these expenses. Find out how much money they are given for the purpose, and what rules they must follow to get the imprest replenished.

Group work

Review the lists of items for which direct cash payment is made, and the lists of staff members with an imprest and the amount of imprest allotted to each.

Discuss the meaning of bills, receipts and vouchers in a petty-cash system.

Identify who grants imprest, who is authorized to spend petty cash, and who is responsible for the imprest. Make comparisons with the allocation system covered in Exercise 49.

Finally, note any of the points discussed here that might improve the functioning of the imprest system.

Exercise 51 (III.4) Managing time: self-assessment

Objective: To be able to monitor and analyse the use of work time.

Individual work

List all the activities and tasks you are expected to perform during a day, as well as all the possible uses of work time you can think of that are not related to work activities (e.g. coffee break, late arrival, etc.) Write these down and then record your use of time over the entire workday, noting precisely the times of beginning and completing each activity, task, or work-related use of time, *as these events occur*. (*Hint*: to ensure accurate recording ask yourself, every 15 minutes or so, "On what activity/task am I engaged just now?" and check whether its starting time, as well as the completion time of the previous task or activity, has been recorded; if not, correct that oversight immediately.)

Activities or tasks that are repeated several times are recorded separately each time; an activity that has been interrupted by another is also recorded separately, from start up to the interruption and from resumption up to the end. (The interrupting activity must also be recorded.)

At the end of the day, calculate and record the exact amount of time spent on each type of activity, task, or work-related use of time. The total should add up to your official number of working hours. If it does not, a new category of time use must be noted, i.e. 'time not accounted for', to make up the difference. Prepare yourself to discuss this use of time with the health team.

Group work

Review and compare the lists of activities, tasks and work-related use of time. Certain groupings may still be made to ensure comparability, e.g. curative, preventive and promotional activities, management, learning and supportive tasks, etc. Similarly, all use of time that is not work-related is called 'non-productive time'. Compare the amount of time spent on the different activities and the unproductive time. Calculate the proportion of unproductive time, and determine how this proportion varies among the health workers. Discuss the significance of these figures for the achievement of health objectives. Decide on possible changes in the use of time to increase productivity.

Exercise 52 (III.4) Observing use of time

Objective: To be able to observe your own and other staff members' use of time, as a means of assessing whether the best use is being made of time and skills.

Individual work

Prepare with a colleague the list of activities and tasks you perform on a workday, as in Exercise 51. While you work through your daily routine your colleague should accompany you and note the time at which you begin and complete each activity or task, including activities that are not work-related, such as coffee breaks, etc. While under observation you should not discuss your use of time. At the end of the workday, calculate together the time spent on each activity or task, as well as the unproductive time. Group the activities and tasks according to the skill they require and calculate the total time spent on each skill-group. Discuss together the adequacy of the observed use of time, given your job description and competence.

Group work

Listen to the presentation of the above findings, and discuss the adequacy of the observed use of time among the different skills. Is work distributed so as to make the best use of the health worker's time and skills towards health objectives? Could redistribution of work improve the use of skills and time? Is delegation needed? If so, what should be delegated and to whom? Do job descriptions need to be revised?

Exercise 53 (III.4) Assessing allocation of time by function

Objective: To be able to assess whether your use of time is appropriate.

Individual work

List your main functions in your health work, and rank them in order of priority according to health objectives and with reference to your job description and work schedule. Each day *for one entire week,* record the time spent (in minutes) on each of the listed functions (in the same way as in Exercises 51 and 52).

At the end of the work week, calculate the total time spent on each function, and draw a diagram showing how you divided the work time between different functions.

Ask yourself, and prepare yourself to discuss with the health team, the following questions:

● Is the observed allocation of work time consistent with the priorities assigned?
● Should anything be changed, and if so how much more or less time should be spent on different functions?

Group work

Listen to the presentations, review the priorities assigned to various functions, and compare the observed use of time, by function, with the priorities set by each health worker.

Calculate also the total time allocated to the various functions by the health team as a whole, and the *proportion* of the total time available spent on these different functions. Discuss this allocation of time in the light of health objectives and priorities for the district, and suggest changes, if needed:

— in objectives and priorities
— in job descriptions
— in work schedules

to ensure that each health worker's allocation of time to the various functions best supports the attainment of health objectives.

Special group work: Use of idle time

Objective: To be able to make the best use of idle time ('non-productive time').

Review the findings of Exercises 51 to 53. Summarize the amount of idle time; analyse when it occurs (in the day, during the week, perhaps seasonally), and whether several health workers have idle time together.

Review the use of work time on various functions, activities and tasks, and decide which of these might usefully be given more time (for instance, continuing education).

Discuss possible activities that could be performed during idle time, either individually or as a whole team; record concrete suggestions such as "coordination meeting during tea-break on Friday".

During the group discussion seek the approval of the medical officer or medical assistant in charge for these suggestions or submit them in writing, seeking a decision on the matter.

Exercise 54 (III.4) Preparing a timetable

Objective: To be able to prepare a health centre timetable.

Individual work

Review your day-to-day functions, activities and tasks as listed in Exercises 51, 52 and 53, and mark those that should be mentioned in the health centre's timetable. Verify that curative, preventive, promotional, support, management, learning, and possibly research functions, activities and tasks are represented in the checklist. Obtain a copy of the current timetable and compare it with your checklist. Does it show specific times for all functions? How much time is allotted to each function? Does the time allotted correspond to the priorities? (If it does not, has time been allotted for exercises such as this one?) Given the health centre's objectives (as discussed in Exercise 53), are some functions given too little time?

Prepare a revised health centre timetable, in accordance with what you regard as a balanced use of time for all staff, and prepare yourself to discuss your proposed revision with the health team.

Group work

Review individual checklists of specific activities that should appear in a health centre timetable. Match the health centre timetable with those checklists, and note any gaps.

Discuss the allocation of time to the various functions and activities, given the priorities and objectives (referring to the conclusions reached in Exercise 52).

Discuss the allocation of time in the light of the perceived needs of staff (time for learning, for staff meetings, etc.)

Then discuss the point of view of patients and others who come to the health centre: does the timetable suit them (times of clinics, meetings, health education sessions, etc.)?

Review critically the individual proposals for revising the timetable, and prepare an agreed revised timetable. For the record, prepare a written justification for each modification; this will help in further revisions.

Special group work: Study of travel time

Objective: To estimate the ratio of travel time to work time in district health work, and to discuss ways of reducing it.

Any health centre whose staff must travel in order to do district work of any kind (family planning, health education, home visiting, supervisory visits, mobile clinics, etc.), whether on foot or by bicycle, bus or motor-vehicle, may be used for this exercise.

List all the district activities of your health centre during a one-month period. Refer to the weekly timetable, and consult the person in charge and other staff to obtain the necessary information.

Ask all staff members who travel:

— how much time (in hours and minutes) they spend travelling in carrying out district activities
— how much time they spend carrying out health work apart from travelling.

Calculate the proportions of time spent in work and in travel by each travelling health worker, using the examples on page 197, and calculate the average for the whole team.

Discuss the following questions:

● Are there other available means of transport that might be tried in an effort to reduce travel time?
● Could travel routes be changed?
● Could health workers visit the village less often and stay longer, or could they stay overnight?
● Could other methods be used to reduce travel time? (See page 197 for suggestions.)

List the group's recommendations for reducing the ratio of travel time to work time.

Exercise 55 (III.4) Preparing schedules

Objective: To write a schedule for follow-up visits to villages for a three-month period.

Schedule for follow-up visits

Health-centre nurses make home visits each week to three outlying villages (A, B and C) for follow-up purposes. Each village is reached by a separate road. A nurse can visit a village, complete her programme and return to the health centre in an afternoon. There are six nurses, and each visits homes on a different afternoon each week.

Individual work

Read pages 201–204.

Using the examples of the schedule on page 202 write a schedule for a three-month period, showing how the nurses could visit each village twice a week. (Disregard the route numbers in the example.)

Examine your final schedule: does it meet the the required criteria:

● Is each of the three villages visited twice a week?
● Are the visits to each village arranged for the same days each week so that the people will know when to expect the nurses?
● Does each staff nurse do home visiting *no more than* one afternoon per week?

Exercise 56 (III.5) Managing work space I

Objective: To be able to organize the available work space to suit the needs of patients and others who use it.

Individual work

Visit in turn each room in the health centre, calling them A, B and C, etc. for later reference.

List the use of space, i.e. the functions, activities and tasks normally performed in each room. As this may vary according to the day and the time of day, record the use of space accordingly. For example:

Room A	Monday	08.00	Sterilization
		09.00	Immunization
		12.00–14.00	Free
		14.00	Health education (maternal and child health)
		17.00	Staff meeting.

Then think of the patients and other people who use these rooms, noting down their number, age groups, sex, special needs. Assess the suitability of the available space in each room for the people involved in the listed functions, activities and tasks: Is *floor space* adequate? Do furniture and equipment leave enough space for people to move? Are *access* (entry) and *exit* through doors easy? Are the seating arrangements suitable? Is the *maintenance* (plastering, painting, decorating) of the working space satisfactory? Is the space *hygienic*: are there spots on the floor or walls, dirt, a foul smell? Are lighting and ventilation adequate? Is the noise level tolerable: does it permit people to communicate? For each of these assessments, note: suitable, needs improvement, unsuitable.

Then think of possible changes for improvement.

Group work

Review and record the suggested changes against specific shortcomings and the descriptions of the groups of patients and others who use the rooms.

For each function, activity or task involving those groups, discuss the suitability of the available space under the following headings:

— floor space
— moving space
— furniture, equipment
— access
— exit
— seating arrangements
— maintenance
    plaster
    paintwork
    decoration

— hygiene
    dirt
    spots
    smells
— lighting
— ventilation.

Note the suggested improvements to the available working space, and discuss how these improvements might be carried out: *who* would do *what* and *when*?

Exercise 57 (III.5) Managing work space II

Objective: To be able to organize the available working space to suit the needs of staff.

Group work

Proceed as in Exercise 56, but focus on staff needs instead of patient needs.

Compare the list of possible improvements in work space suggested to meet the needs of patients and staff. Where conflicting improvements are suggested, try to resolve them by discussion. Then confirm the proposed improvement programmes (*who, what, when?*) and discuss priorities in implementation, beginning with all changes that do not require additional expenditure.

Record these suggestions and recommendations for consideration by the medical officer or medical assistant in charge.

Exercise 58 (III.5) Managing hygiene in a health facility

Objective: To be able to keep the work space in optimal hygienic condition.

Individual work

Review the list of defects in hygiene compiled in Exercises 56 and 57, and record them on separate sheets, room by room, function by function, according to how they affect patients, staff, or both.

Analyse each unhygienic condition to determine its main cause (e.g. building design, maintenance, behaviour of patients and others, work organization, etc.). Record these systematically and determine the most common causes of the listed unhygienic conditions. Starting with the most common causes, suggest specific remedial measures — one or two for each defective room.

Think of *who* should plan, execute, or supervise remedial measures, and outline a programme for introducing these measures over, say, a three-month period.

Group work

Review the list of unhygienic conditions. Analyse the suggested causes, note the causes that are most common and place them in priority order according to the feasibility of remedying them.

Programme the priority remedial measures to be introduced over the next three months. Verify (e.g. in the staff job descriptions) whose responsibility it is to plan, execute, and supervise these measures. Assign to the staff present the various tasks involved in the improvement programme.

Record conclusions, and assignments, for submission to the person in charge of the health facility.

Exercise 59 (III.5) Work-flow arrangements

Objective: To be able to recognize signs of poor working arrangements that affect the movement of outpatients through the health centre.

Individual work

The health worker in charge of patient registration gives each outpatient on arrival a slip of paper showing the exact time of entering the waiting area (e.g. WAIT: 7.50 h.) Patients are told to show the slip to all staff members who interview, examine or treat them and to return it to the health worker they meet last. Whenever a patient moves from one station to the next, the health worker in the station records on the patient's slip the activity, and its starting and completion time (e.g. LAB: 3.15h/3.22 h). Patients are always told precisely where to go next.

The health worker at the last station visited by a patient (e.g. pharmacy, or health education) retains the slip, with the recorded starting and completion times.

If patients return to the waiting area between two stations, the registration clerk records the time spent there (e.g. WAIT: 8.25/8.50); if they stay in the waiting area after they have finished, the time spent there is also recorded.

Group work

Collect all patients' slips for the day and tabulate the findings on a chalkboard, patient by patient. For each patient and each station record:

— the *sequence* in which the patient visited the various stations (flow)
— the *time* spent in each station (processing time).

Collate the information on *flow*, note the most common sequences, and calculate the proportion of patients following the most common flow patterns.

Collate the information on time spent in each station, underline the shortest and longest recorded time, and calculate the *mean time* spent in each station, including the waiting-room. Record the most common flow patterns and discuss the possible reasons for different sequences. Could the flow be standardized or rationalized?

Compare the mean time spent in various stations with the mean total time, and discuss the possible reasons for the differences observed.

Calculate the proportion of mean total time spent in the waiting area, and discuss why so much time should be spent waiting compared with the time spent on services.

Work out changes in the use of space that might reduce the time taken for patients to go through the process. Suggest other possible changes that might contribute to improving the flow.

> **NOW FILL IN**
> **THE EVALUATION SHEET**
> **THAT FOLLOWS**

Evaluation of Part III

On the 0 to 5 scale, mark with a tick (✓) the extent of your agreement with the following statements:

Reading material is:
    relevant to my work   0--/--/--/--/--/--5
    useful for my work   0--/--/--/--/--/--5
    difficult to understand   0--/--/--/--/--/--5
    too time-consuming   0--/--/--/--/--/--5

Individual exercises are:
    relevant to the subject   0--/--/--/--/--/--5
    useful as means of learning   0--/--/--/--/--/--5
    difficult to perform   0--/--/--/--/--/--5
    too time-consuming   0--/--/--/--/--/--5

Group exercises are:
    relevant to the team's work   0--/--/--/--/--/--5
    useful for the team's work   0--/--/--/--/--/--5
    difficult to perform   0--/--/--/--/--/--5
    too time-consuming   0--/--/--/--/--/--5

I have acquired:
    new knowledge   0--/--/--/--/--/--5
    new attitudes   0--/--/--/--/--/--5
    new skills   0--/--/--/--/--/--5

PART IV

Managing primary health care services

Introduction

A health worker is responsible for the health care of a population in a geographical area. This area may be as small as a village or as large as a district but, whether small or large, there are always problems to be overcome in delivering health care.

In Part IV the concepts of management outlined in Parts I, II and III are applied to the health care of a community. The health worker with management duties must work closely with the community in planning and implementing the health programme; therefore, before discussing management, it is necessary to consider in more detail:

— how to manage primary health care in the community, and
— how to increase health coverage by developing community self-help programmes.

Working in the community

The various components of the health system discussed in Part III (e.g. money, time, people, and equipment) are resources that enable health workers to apply their skills and cooperate with communities in improving and maintaining acceptable levels of health care.

The health worker attached to a health centre has a special responsibility to support the village health worker and, at the same time, to be the link between that worker and the central or regional level of the health service.

The newly appointed health worker will almost always have management functions, and must therefore get to know the people and find out as much as possible about their problems and needs, from other health workers in the district and from community leaders. Many of the problems may not seem to be health problems but most, like poor housing and malnutrition, will be causes of, or associated with, health problems. People will not become or remain healthy until these problems are dealt with. Such problems call for cooperation between the health sector and other sectors, such as education or agriculture; others can be solved by the people themselves with help and suggestions from health workers.

Most countries have a national health plan or a number of national programmes such as maternal and child health and control of communicable disease (e.g. leprosy, tuberculosis). The ministry of health sets general policy and specifies the general objectives of programmes that have to be implemented at the middle and primary levels. These general objectives must be broken down into intermediate objectives and targets. For example, a national objective may be to eradicate poliomyelitis. A programme objective may be to reduce the incidence of paralytic poliomyelitis by 50%, and a target may be "to immunize all children under two years of age, that is three million children, against poliomyelitis in the two years from 1.1.1993 to 1.1.1995". At the district level the target is broken down to the number of children under two years in a particular district, which may be 5000. At the primary level, the figure of 5000 must be broken down to cover several villages, perhaps 1000 children in one village, 500 children in another and so on until the area is covered. Each primary health worker will have a small target in a small area. The total of several small areas will make up the 5000 children to be immunized in the district.

Increasing health coverage

In many countries large numbers of families still have no access to health care or are not covered by the health system. How can one primary health worker in a village provide health care for many people, especially those who live more than 10 to 20 km away? One way is to work with communities and use community resources so that, for a number of tasks, communities can take care of themselves, with support from the community health worker who visits them from time to time. The village people will send the sick or those who need more skilled care and advice to the community health worker or the nurse at the dispensary or health centre.

The health worker in the management role increases health coverage by training and supporting community health workers and in other ways extending health coverage of the public.

Example: Increasing health coverage in a community

Maria, the community health worker at San Canto, knows that many young children are undernourished. She talks to people in the community and learns that many women have stopped breast-feeding their babies because powdered milk is available and "is very good for babies". However, Maria knows that no milk is as good as breast milk for babies. She also knows that the mothers do not have the necessary knowledge or the hygienic conditions to prepare powdered milk properly. The mixture may be contaminated with dust and flies, or be too weak or too strong, so that the babies get diarrhoea and lose weight.

Maria wants to change this and encourage women to breast-feed, but she is alone. She discusses the problem with her supervisor, who helps her to make a decision. After much thought Maria visits the three communities for which she is responsible and talks with the community leaders. They introduce her to women in the community who are breast-feeding their babies successfully. Maria talks with the women and, after discussion, each community chooses a leader from among these women. Maria works with the women leaders, who learn how to answer questions, how to listen, how to use a teaching aid and how to make up stories, so that they can teach others.

The women leaders then invite pregnant women and mothers with sick babies to come for a discussion. For the first few talks Maria joins the group, helping the women leaders in their task of explaining and teaching why breast-feeding is so valuable and how long it should continue.

As time goes by, changes occur: more women breast-feed their babies. Meanwhile the women leaders, with Maria's help, learn more about child feeding and health care, simple first aid, signs of illness and certain treatments. They teach these things to other people.

From this small beginning, health care is extended to many families. The people would not have got help if they had had to rely on the health worker alone, and Maria could not have done so much without the community's help. Now she can give more time to sick people, organize immunization campaigns, and provide antenatal care for pregnant women. The women leaders refer people to Maria if they need more specialized care.

CHAPTER 1

Planning health activities

Introduction: The planning function

In Part I the principle of management by objectives was seen to be very closely related to the planning function of management. However, other principles discussed there also concern this function. The principle of division of labour has a direct bearing on the planning and organization of manpower. A good plan should make clear the tasks to be performed and the personnel to be assigned to perform them. Similarly the principle of economizing on scarce resources concerns planning, as determining resource needs and preparing budgets are important aspects of planning. The reader may pause and review the other principles in Part I to see which of them, if any, relate to the planning function.

What, then, is the planning function of management? One way to consider it is: planning is an attempt to answer questions *before* they actually arise, anticipating as many implementation decisions as possible by foreseeing possible problems, and deriving principles and setting rules for solving them. Planning therefore includes the specification of evaluation criteria, rules, norms, etc. that will be used in implementation decisions.

The reader may appreciate the kinds of *decision* involved in planning, by imagining an intended journey. A traveller would have to decide on:

— destination
— route
— mode of transport, accommodation
— how to avoid or overcome possible obstacles or difficulties
— equipment, clothing
— cost of travel and how much he or she can afford to pay
— day-by-day schedule.

Similarly, a planner will have to decide on:

— the objectives of what is being planned
— the approach, or strategy, for reaching the objectives
— the activities (e.g. services) required to achieve the objectives
— the obstacles that may hamper activities
— the resources to be used
— the cost of activities
— the detailed scheduling of implementation.

To determine more precisely the types of decision to be made in each of these areas, it is useful to go through the following questions: why?, what?, which?, who?, where?, how?, how much? and when?, and to apply them to the three principal areas of planning, namely:

— objectives
— activities
— resources.

The following brief review makes it clear that the planning function must be a collective undertaking. No one 'manager' could undertake all the analysis, design and quantification necessary for planning the work of a health team. Realistic planning requires the cooperation of all those who have the necessary information, knowledge and powers of decision. This stresses once again that management is a shared responsibility, and that each member of the team has a share of this responsibility.

Planning decisions about objectives

What?
Which?
Why?
Who?
Where?
How much?

The first planning decision is to determine what problems there are and which of them merit priority attention. A problem may be a gap between what is and what could be, or an obstacle to bridging such a gap. The planner must also decide who is at risk from the problem, or is exposed to or affected by it, where those at risk live and work, their social class, and the 'catchment area' where they can be reached. The most important planning decision is the extent to which it is intended to reduce the problem, and the target time for achieving the reduction. In short, the planning function is to analyse the problems and decide on the changes to be made.

Planning decisions about activities

What?
Which?
Whom?
How much?
How?
By whom?

The first decision concerns the activities that are needed, perhaps under the broad headings of service, development and support activities. For each activity, the target individuals, group or population at whom the activity is directed must be decided. (These are not necessarily the people directly affected by the problem; for example, mothers may be educated about child nutrition.) Then a decision is needed about the amounts of each type of activity required to reach the target group, for example one, two or three visits. Often there is a choice of ways of performing the activities: there may be a variety of possible techniques, methods and institutional frameworks. A decision must be made about the right approach in the particular circumstances. Further decisions concern timing, sequence, frequency, location of activities, and assignment of tasks and responsibilities to individual members of the health team. In short, the planning function entails designing in detail the activities of the team.

Planning decisions about resources

Which?
How much?
Where?

Decisions about resources differ from those concerning objectives and activities in being mainly quantitative. As soon as the nature of the resources required — staff,

When?
From where?
Who?

equipment, supplies, etc. — has been determined, decisions will be made about the necessary amounts of each resource. This will enable costs to be estimated, and thus decisions to be made about budget. Logistic considerations will help in deciding where the resources needed to implement the specified activities should come from and be sent. In particular, some decision will be needed about where funds will come from, i.e. financing arrangements in which various sources of funds, from communities to external agencies, may contribute varying proportions of the budget. This planning function is therefore concerned with the specification and quantification of resources.

Summary

- **The planning function of management in a health team deals mainly with decisions about objectives, activities and resources, by systematically considering what, which, where, when, how much, and how the team will perform.**
- **Because of its complexity, planning is best shared by all team members and by representatives of the community.**

Planning health activities step by step

Planning begins as an idea or in response to attention being drawn to a particular situation. It can take place at any level of a health system. Usually, however, the ministry of health lays down the general policies and guidelines of the system. The role of the health team is then to interpret policies at local level, plan their implementation, and ensure that they are implemented.

During routine work, planning takes place continually. Planning methods can be applied to a large programme such as a national malaria programme or to a small one such as health education of a single patient.

This chapter focuses on five planning steps:

Step 1	Looking at the situation
Step 2	Recognizing problems
Step 3	Setting objectives
Step 4	Reviewing obstacles
Step 5	Scheduling the activities

Step 1: Looking at the situation

Learning objectives

After studying Step 1 and doing Exercise 60 on page 369, the health worker should be able to:

— **gather information from the community**

— **extract information from records**

— **tabulate cumulative data**

— **analyse and interpret information**

— **review existing health work**

— **collect information on resources.**

Sources of information

For purposes of planning primary health care services, information is needed about:

— the community (population, births and deaths, age groups, housing, schools, leaders, organization, etc.)
— health, diseases and illnesses
— organization of the health service
— health staff
— community resources.

Some of this information may be obtained from various sectors other than health, such as education and agriculture. Much of it may be obtained from records and reports. This is usually formal (or official, or published) information.

Information may be obtained informally from the community rather than from official sources, and is probably the most useful for planning health programmes. Much can be learnt from discussions with different groups—community leaders, teachers, traditional health workers, women's groups. Such people can indicate a community's needs and often uncover the underlying cause of a problem when it is not apparent to the health worker. For example, when mothers of young children, despite sustained interest in nutrition education, fail to practise what they have learned, the reason may be that the grandmothers, who are often heads of households, have a strong traditional approach to the rearing and feeding of children.

The following table shows the types and sources of the information that may usefully be collected about a community and its health problems and needs:

Types and sources of information and methods of collection

Types	Source and method
On people's health	*Community*
Why problems have occurred The kinds of traditional health care available Attitudes and customs concerning health and illness	Listening and observing in the community Talking with people
On health work being done	
What the people feel about the work What the people feel they need	Listening to what people say, particularly the leaders Talking with other community development workers
On the community	
Attitudes and customs relating to matters other than health, e.g. communication between leaders and people. Who are the leaders? Who makes decisions and how are decisions reached? Are there traditional health workers such as birth attendants, healers, medicine-men? Other health or health-related agencies	Listening to and talking with people Reading material Talking with other health and development workers Talking with teachers and religious leaders
Geographical features Transport facilities Public facilities: water, sanitation, markets, schools, farming, food production Source of water	Map of area
To identify people	*Records*
Name, age, sex, address	Registration cards Health centre records Community survey Household survey
On people's health	
Kinds of health problem and when they occurred Number of pregnant women attending antenatal clinics	Monthly reports Outpatient records Clinic records

Types	Source and method
Number of births each month or each year (live and still births) and sex	Clinic records or survey of children under one year in the community
Number of maternal deaths associated with pregnancy and childbirth in past year	Clinic records or direct questioning in the villages
Number of deaths by sex, age and presumed cause	Possibly, health centre records, or records of community officials
On health work being done	
Number of people seen each month, and for what reasons	Monthly reports
Treatment given, kinds of health problem	
Special campaigns held	
On materials used for health work	
Drugs supplied	Stock ledgers and inventory
Drugs used	
Other supplies	
Estimate of supplies needed for a period of time	
On health workers	
Needs for training	Supervisory checklist for visits to the community
Quality of work	
Relations with community and other agencies	
Use of resources	

Collecting baseline information on the community

Baseline information often needs to be collected to decide what kinds of health activity are needed and to calculate the number of people who should receive different kinds of health service. It also enables progress to be measured at intervals.

Such baseline information would include:

— number of people and distribution by sex
— distribution by age groups (years), 0–1, 1–5, 5–9, 10–14, 15–24, 25–34 .... 65+
— the principal occupations
— the typical composition of a family
— number of births in the community in the past year
— number of stillbirths or deaths of children under one year in the past year
— probable causes of deaths

— most common diseases
— whom people call or consult when they are sick
— topography (geographical features) of the area
— water supply sources
— excreta disposal practices
— foods available and used.

This information may be collected in different ways. Village leaders can provide some of it, but a household survey may be necessary to find out all that is needed.

By conducting interviews in all, or in a sample of, households, a survey may be made of, for example, number of people in each house or, in areas with many houses, in every fourth or fifth house. Health workers often need the assistance of village volunteers in collecting information. They must be told why and how the survey is being done, and what information to collect. The village leader may advise on the choice of volunteers. It is generally necessary to prepare a survey questionnaire. An example of a survey form is shown below:

Household survey

Date: **Investigator:**

1. Place ....

(District)   (Village)   (Road)   (House no.)

2. Composition of household

Names of household members	Age	Sex	Principal occupation

3. Important events during previous year

Births Date	Name	Live/still	Deaths Date	Name	Probable cause

4. Status of head of household

Degree of literacy:

Education (schooling):
None ( ) Less than 3 years ( ) 3–6 years ( )   7 years or more ( )

Occupation:
Agriculture ( )   Craft   ( )   Industry   ( )   Services   ( )

Income:
No cash   ( )   Cash   ( )   If cash, amount . . . .

Ownership:
House ( )   Land   ( )   (. . . . . . hectares)   Animals (. . . . .)
Tools (. . . . .)

5. Environment

House:
Area . . . . m²   Wall material . . . .
Roof material . . . . No. of openings . . . . .

Water:
Daily consumption . . . . . litres   Source . . . .
Storage facilities . . . . Disposal facilities . . . .

6. Health information

6.1 Children

Names of children under 5 years (M/F)	Height	Weight	Arm circumference

6.2 Illness in the household in the previous year

Date	Name	Main symptoms	Duration

6.3 Disabilities at time of survey

Name	Nature of disability	Duration (years)

6.4 Opinion on priority health problems in the community

6.5 Care of sick members of household

Home care   (   )   Outside help   (   )   From whom? . . . .

6.6 Care of pregnant women

Service used:
Prenatal   (   )   Delivery   (   )   Postnatal   (   )
Provided by:
Midwife   (   )   Traditional birth attendant   (   )   Other   (   )

6.7 Infant and child feeding

Duration of breast-feeding: . . . .

Age at introduction of: cereals . . . .   months
fruit/vegetables. . . . .   months
fish/meat . . . .   months
adult food. . . . .   months

6.8 Contraceptive practices

Name	Method	Since (date)

6.9 Health consultations in previous year

Date	Name	Place	Result	Comment

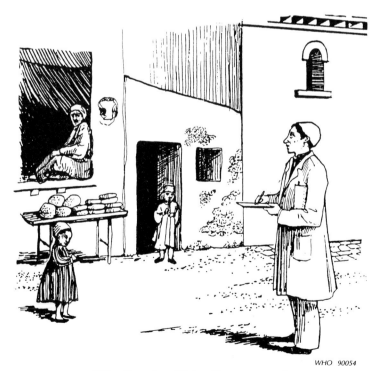

WHO 90054

"Who lives here?" (making a survey)

Information about available resources

Information about resources is essential. A resource may be anybody or anything that can be used to carry out activities to achieve an objective.

When choosing a course of action, all types of community and health service resources must be considered systematically, one by one. The main types are the following:

- People: trained people, skilled people, or others who are involved in providing health care services.
- Buildings, e.g. dispensaries, health centres, rural hospitals.
- Equipment, material, transport.
- Information: books and manuals, records and reports, community studies, surveys.
- Social and environmental factors: public opinion, government support, technical resources (e.g. electricity), climate.
- Money: needed to obtain other resources (such as to purchase drugs).
- Time: for instance, times at which people are most likely to participate in health programmes.

Collecting information to explain the cause of a problem

Information may also have to be collected to help in understanding why a particular problem has occurred. Thus, an investigation may be needed to determine why the monthly report shows an increase in the incidence of diarrhoea. Questions such as the following might need to be considered:

- Do the people understand the necessity for good hygiene and sanitation?
- Are there attitudes and customs that could cause the problems?
- Is the water supply safe? If not, why not?
- Are the people using the latrines that have been built? If not, why not?

Answers will give information that may lead to a fuller or more accurate interpretation of the data found in records.

From information gathered, the health worker can plan better ways to solve problems or to modify programmes.

Looking at the health work being done

It is useful to make a list of targets previously set and to check which have been achieved (e.g. a targeted number of children immunized) and which have not. This also helps in learning about the obstacles and difficulties encountered in trying to reach targets. At times there may be no information about the achievement of targets, because the basic records are not available or reliable: this in itself is also important information.

The community's opinions about health work should be noted. Are the people participating fully in certain programmes? Are they satisfied with the work being done? Are they applying what they learn and what the health worker teaches? What are the obstacles? Can such obstacles be removed or reduced? Should targets be changed?

Tabulating cumulative information

To review health work, it is useful to arrange information in the form of a table.

Example: Target achievement review table

Programme	Target met?	Obstacles

MCH: antenatal care
      deliveries
	No
	Yes
		Lack of transport to
		     mountainous area

Communicable disease
    control: diarrhoea
	Latrines? No
	Health education
	    programme? Yes
	Water?
		Attitudes of village people
		
		(Data not available)

```
REVIEW INFORMATION
```

Information collected daily can be accumulated by adding the data for each month throughout the year. In this way a health worker can see how each programme is progressing, and where and why targets are not being met. This information is very useful in making the health plan for the following year.

Analysing information

It is not enough simply to collect information. The information must also be analysed and 'digested'.

Information must be selected so that only what is *useful* is considered. It should be arranged in such a way that it can be compared with other information (standardized), and recorded so that it can be remembered, found again when needed, and communicated to others who need it.

Summary — Step 1

- **Look at the whole situation**
- **Understand the community**
- **Look at existing health services**
- **Study the resources**
- **Analyse the causes of problems**
- **Record and tabulate findings**

Step 2: Recognizing important problems

Learning objectives

After studying Step 2 and doing Exercise 61 on page 370, the health worker should be able to:

— recognize and list the problems that exist in the community

— select important problems according to criteria

— recognize problems that are the responsibility of other agencies outside the health service.

What is a problem?

Two useful definitions of a problem are the following:

● A problem is a difficulty or obstacle seen to exist between a present situation and a desired future objective.

● A problem is a perceived gap between what is and what should be.

It must be recognized that different people perceive problems differently.

Example:

A village has a contaminated water supply, which may be resulting in outbreaks of diarrhoea.

If the villagers do not recognize that the water is contaminated or that it is responsible for diarrhoea, they will not perceive contamination of the water supply and the resulting diarrhoea as a problem.

But the health worker sees or perceives the gap between what is and what could be. To the health worker, this gap is a problem.

A problem must be clearly defined, otherwise any attempted solution may be the wrong one. Many health problems have several causes. It is easy to mistake a cause for a problem; then one cause may be removed without

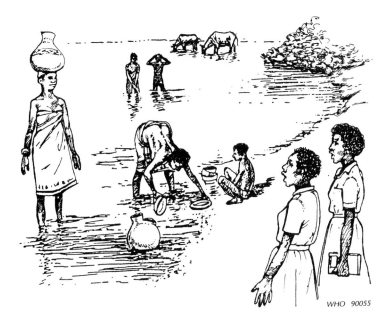

A 'problem' as seen by a health worker

WHO 90055

solving the problem. Consider the following:

1) Many people have diarrhoea.
2) The well-water is contaminated.
3) There are too many flies.
4) Sanitation is poor.
5) The people lack health education.

Which is the health problem?

The health *problem* is "many people have diarrhoea". Statements 2, 3, 4 and 5 are possible *causes* of the problem.

If the problem is stated as "sanitation is poor", and the effort to solve the problem is concerned only with improved sanitation, the diarrhoea will not disappear. It may still be spread by flies or contaminated water and by the unhealthy behaviour of the people.

In solving a problem:

— analyse and define what the problem is
— find all its possible causes
— look for ways to remove the causes.

Selecting important problems

To select important problems it is useful to group all the problems under the following headings:

- *Diseases or health problems*, e.g.

  Malaria
  Malnutrition
  Respiratory diseases
  Diarrhoea

- *Health service problems*, e.g.

  Insufficient drugs
  Lack of qualified personnel
  Difficulty in visiting outlying areas

- *Community problems*, e.g.

  Inadequate water supply
  No primary education
  People have to go a long way for health care
  Poor harvest two years running
  Male population leaving the land to work in industry

The health worker is always faced with more than one problem at a time and cannot solve all of them at once. The problems must be studied and the most important given priority, i.e. these problems will be tackled first. Resources will be used mainly for these problems.

When attempting to select priority problems it is important to look carefully for the real causes, especially for purposes of planning health interventions. Many health problems could best be cured by more and better food, clean water, education, and solid, safe housing. When seeking information the health worker must also look outside the health field.

One way to determine problem priorities is to set and apply selection criteria. A criterion is a principle or a standard by which something can be measured or judged. A set of criteria may be established as a *checklist* such as the following:

Does the problem:

— affect large numbers of people, e.g. malaria, AIDS (acquired immuno-deficiency syndrome), leprosy?

— cause high infant mortality, e.g. malnutrition, neonatal tetanus?
— affect maternal health, e.g. complications of pregnancy, multiple pregnancies, postpartum haemorrhage?
— affect children and young people, e.g. tuberculosis, road accidents, accidents in the home?
— cause chronic conditions and handicap, e.g. blindness, trachoma, poliomyelitis?
— affect rural development, e.g. river blindness, sleeping sickness?
— cause great concern to the whole community?

If the answer to any of the above questions is YES, the problem is one that should be given priority.

A problem also may receive priority attention if there is a simple way to deal with it.

Example: A list of community problems

After reviewing all the information available, a number of different kinds of problem will emerge. A typical list might read as follows:

Diseases or health problems

Malaria
Respiratory infections
Diarrhoea
Complications of pregnancy and labour
Eye infections
Insect and snake bites
Low birth weight of infants
AIDS
Leprosy
Tuberculosis
Hepatitis
Skin infections
Ear infections
Malnutrition
(and so on, according to the area).

Communications

Bad roads
Seasonal bad weather
Avalanches
Inadequate transport
Flooding

Health services

Health personnel do not go out to the community
Lack of material for dressings and treatments
Insufficient staff
Insufficient drugs
Inadequate working conditions
Lack of transport

Other problems affecting health

Illiteracy
Lack of sanitation
Contaminated water supply
Bad and overcrowded housing
Rodents and other animals roaming freely
Drought
Unemployment

To discover which of these are priority problems the selection criteria on pages 284–285 should be applied; the more important problems will become obvious, for instance:

Health problems

Complications of labour
Low birth weight of infants
Malnutrition

Health service problems

Too few visits to the community
Lack of transport.

Community problems

Lack of sanitation.

Many problems are outside the scope of the health sector but they must be considered because they affect health. The health worker can set health education of the people as a priority, to inform them about these problems and teach them how to prevent and overcome them. This may mean cooperating with the schoolteacher, or with the literacy programme, to prepare material to help people learn about health at the same time as they learn to read.

Contaminated water or lack of water is not a problem that health workers can tackle alone. They can get in touch with the responsible people and cooperate with them, and must consider this in making work plans. A plan may provide for, e.g. education of, and participation with, the community in a latrine-building programme or in efforts to conserve water in the home.

Example: The district of Vosok

Nurse-midwife Shireen has collected and analysed information in the district of Vosok. She notes that complications of pregnancy and delivery are high on the list of the people's concerns. She knows that the government is also concerned about the number of women dying during or after childbirth, as well as about the number of children born dead or dying soon after birth. As a result, the national objective to reduce maternal mortality by providing antenatal care and increasing the health coverage of pregnant women is being emphasized throughout the country.

In Vosok, Shireen notes that women are poorly educated and that pregnant women do not go for health care, and that these difficulties are associated with the high maternal mortality.

After deciding that complications of pregnancy and delivery are priority problems in her district, nurse-midwife Shireen organizes an antenatal programme.

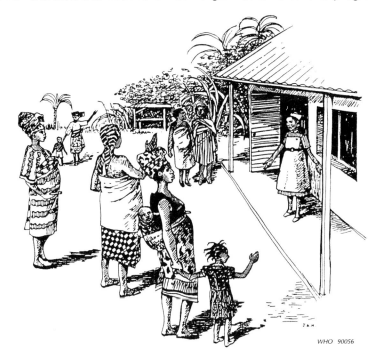

WHO 90056

Encouraging women to have antenatal care

Summary — Step 2

There should be a list of the important problems of the community

- **clearly defined**
- **with possible causes**
- **in order of importance.**

Step 3: Setting objectives

Learning objectives

After studying Step 3, the health worker should be able to:

— **set objectives that are relevant, feasible, measurable and observable**

— **write programme objectives**

— **specify measurable targets.**

After priority problems have been selected, the next step is to decide how far the problems can be reduced or whether they can be solved. Many health problems cannot be solved quickly. They need several combined activities to deal with them, because they concern people.

Setting objectives is a positive step towards improving health. An objective states a definite expected result. Often, care services are provided year after year but little or no improvement is seen in the community's health, because the health activities have had no clear objectives. By setting objectives, what is done can be continuously assessed and, at the end of a determined period, can be evaluated, i.e. the achievements of the programme can be measured and a judgement made about its value, after which changes can be made to improve it.

An objective may be defined as follows:

● An objective is the intended result of a successful programme or activity.

There are two important reasons for setting objectives. The first is that a clear objective is essential to a definite plan. If you say "I am going East", no definite travel plans can be made. But if you say "I am going to Shanghai", a travel plan can be drawn up, e.g. bus from village to town, train from town to port, boat from port to Shanghai.

You may say "we shall improve health", but no definite plan can be made from that. But if you say "we shall ensure access to health care for the total population by 1995", a plan can be drawn up to try to achieve that goal. Long-term objectives, such as to control or eradicate a communicable disease — measles or poliomyelitis for instance — or to reduce the infant mortality rate, require that a number of intermediate objectives, necessary to achieve the main objective, be stated. Short-term objectives to be achieved by a specific date as a step towards a long-term objective are called 'operational targets'.

The second reason for setting objectives is to enable results to be evaluated. When a programme has no stated or known objective, its outcome cannot be evaluated. Thus, if the objective of a child health programme is to reduce infant mortality by a specific proportion within a given period, evaluation of the programme necessitates measuring the degree of reduction achieved within the determined period. If the objective is to reduce the number of cases of measles by 50% by 1995, the result can be quantified as the number of cases of measles in the population in 1995 compared with the number in each of the previous five years.

Objectives are usually time-limited, i.e. to be achieved in a certain number of weeks, months or years.

Characteristics of useful objectives

Objectives must satisfy certain criteria: they must be relevant, feasible, and observable or measurable.

An objective is *relevant* if it either fits in with general health policy or relates to the problem to be solved or reduced.

An objective is *feasible* if it can be achieved, i.e. if the resources are available and the obstacles can be overcome.

An objective is *observable* when its achievement can be clearly seen or measured. If a building is erected or a worker is trained in a new skill, this is a result that can be seen.

An objective is *measurable* when the outcome or result can be stated in numbers. For example, "malnutrition will be reduced to 1%" is measurable; "all newborn babies in the Maternity Unit will be vaccinated with BCG" is measurable — at the end of the year the number of babies born and the number vaccinated can be compared, i.e. progress towards achieving the objective can be measured.

Objectives may be stated at different levels of the health system

The following is an example of an objective set by a ministry of health at national level:

- "At the end of 5 years, less than 4% of children under three years of age will be undernourished (below 60% weight for age on standard growth chart)."

At the district level, objectives are expressed as a number of operational targets. The following are examples of operational targets and their corresponding activities:

- To discover children of 0–3 years of age with malnutrition, according to stated nutritional criteria (the villages and the number of children to be covered should be listed).
- To train village health workers to recognize malnutrition according to criteria (the number of village health workers to be trained should be stated).
- To organize a (definite) number of training sessions.
- To provide care to malnourished children according to standard instructions[1] (the quality of care can be assessed).

At village level the operational targets of a primary health care worker would be:

- To register all newborn babies.
- To discover among the child population of 0–3 years of age all children with malnutrition (according to the specified criteria).
- To provide care to the malnourished children according to the standard instructions.[1]

In the following two examples, some objectives are examined against a checklist of questions to find out whether they are relevant, feasible, observable and/or measurable.

---

[1] Standard instructions are expressed as *activities* of the programme, i.e. what health workers should do. The results can be evaluated at intervals to judge progress and at the end of a plan period, e.g. after five years, to see whether or to what extent the objective has been achieved.

Example 1: Checking objectives against criteria

● "An improved general nutritional level in District X by 1995."

Is this relevant?	Yes, if there is known to be a definite problem of undernutrition.
Is this feasible?	Yes, if it is based on knowledge of the local conditions, and if resources are available or can be obtained.
Is this observable?	No, not until "nutritional level" has been defined in a way that can be observed, for example by measuring upper arm circumference (in centimetres).

● "To reduce the transmission rate of hookworm in District Y by next year."

Is this relevant?	Yes, if the condition is widespread and causes anaemia.
Is this feasible?	No. The time stated (next year) is too short for the many operational targets (sanitation and educational work) that would be necessary.
Is this observable?	Yes, if the present transmission rate is known.
Is this measurable?	No, not until the proposed reduction of transmission is stated in numbers or as a percentage.

Example 2: Setting a measurable target

An objective is stated as "to provide more pregnant women with antenatal and ordinary medical care". The number or proportion of pregnant women who will receive antenatal care in a specified time may be stated as the target. Setting such a measurable operational target enables the result of an activity to be evaluated. The target can therefore be stated as "to provide 60% of pregnant women in the district with antenatal care during the current year". The total expected number of pregnant women in a village in one year can be determined by using the crude birth rate for the country, if this is available. The health worker in charge learns from her supervisor that the crude birth rate is 40/1000.[1] She

---

[1] If the birth rate for the country is not known, an estimate of the total number of expected pregnancies in a village for one year can be made by checking the number of births in the village during the previous year, as reported in the village survey. This can be a rough estimate for immediate use.

For future years a health worker in charge of the area should arrange for all births in the village to be reported, either to the village leader or to the village health worker. In this way, the number of births each year for a five-year period could be added and the total divided by five. This would provide a more accurate picture of the average number of expected births each year.

knows from the village survey report that the population of the village is 3200. She uses the following formula to determine the expected number of births:

Population × birth rate = number of expected births

$$3200 \times \frac{40}{1000} = 128 \text{ expected births}$$

(Of course, there will always be more pregnancies than births because some pregnancies will not end in childbirth.)

She then considers the resources, including health workers and traditional birth attendants, available for the programme and estimates that she can reach in a year the 77 pregnant women who are the target for the programme (60%).

A MEASURABLE TARGET HAS BEEN SET

Setting such targets for programmes enables a health worker to tell from monthly reports how well a programme is progressing during the year and to evaluate it at the end of the year.

Example: Setting objectives in the district of Vosok

Nurse-midwife Shireen has reviewed her choice of objective, "to provide as many pregnant women as possible with antenatal care".

- The community expresses a great need for maternal care.
- There are many maternal and neonatal deaths, which makes maternal care a priority health problem.
- Increasing maternal health coverage is a national priority.
- Substantial increase in coverage is practicable though difficult.
- Obstacles may be overcome with community participation.

So that she can plan and organize the work and measure the achievement, Shireen sets a target: "to provide 60% of the expected number of pregnant mothers in sector A with antenatal care during the year 1993".

Summary — Step 3

● **An objective is the intended result or achievement of a programme or activity.**

● **Objectives should be relevant, feasible, observable, and measurable.**

● **Objectives are essential for making plans and for evaluating results.**

● **Operational targets are steps towards an objective; they refer to specified activities, populations and periods.**

● **The health team sets its own operational targets towards national objectives.**

Step 4: Reviewing obstacles and limitations

Learning objectives

After studying Step 4 and doing Exercise 62 on page 370, the health worker should be able to:

— recognize obstacles to the achievement of targets

— analyse ways of overcoming obstacles

— recognize limitations that cannot be removed.

After objectives have been set, the questions "Are there any reasons why these objectives could not be attained? Are there limitations or obstacles in the way?" must be asked.

Types of obstacles and limitations

The *limitations* of an activity may be simply the shortage of *resources* discovered during a review of resources.

For example:

- *People* are not interested, or they feel they have other more important needs, or there are no trained or skilled people to perform certain activities.
- *Equipment* is not available or is too expensive.
- *Information* is hard to find: there are no books, and statistics are not available.
- *Money* cannot be raised from local communities.
- *Time*: staff do not have enough time to do all they are expected to do.

There may be special *environmental obstacles*. When making a plan the environment should be reviewed to see whether it presents any special difficulties, such as:

- *Geographical features*, which would be important for building roads, marketing goods, or transporting patients to hospital; for instance, mountains, rivers and lakes may be serious obstacles to delivering an adequate health service in some areas.

- *Climate*, which may influence types of building, transport, growth of vegetables, nature of health problems, etc.
- *Technical difficulties* related to the technical development of the society; for instance, an electric centrifuge is useless in a health centre where there is no electricity.
- *Social factors*, which are the most serious obstacles: there may be customs or taboos that operate against the plan, people may be prejudiced against new ideas, or there may be laws or regulations (good or bad) that prevent certain activities.

Analysing the obstacles

A simple method of analysing obstacles is to list the objectives, write down the obstacles and limitations for each one and show them under three headings, as follows:

- *Obstacles that can be removed*, i.e. a solution may be found. For example: "to provide and improve maternity care". The obstacle: a shortage of qualified midwives. The suggested solution is to train traditional birth attendants and have supervision provided by midwives.
- *Obstacles that can be modified or reduced*. For example: a group of villages want their children to be educated. They set as targets "to build a school and recruit a teacher". They find their resources are insufficient, so instead of a schoolhouse they build a house that may attract a teacher to come to a rural area. A teacher can teach without a school building, but a building, however well equipped, is useless without a teacher.
- *Obstacles that cannot be removed or reduced*. Most people have a more or less fixed income, at least for long periods of time. People can budget in a better way, use money differently, and look for bargains, but the income is unchanged and living must be adjusted to it. In health planning, one objective must sometimes be replaced by another that needs fewer resources. For example, if it is planned to employ a midwife-supervisor and none is available, the goal may be changed so as to have an experienced and trained traditional birth attendant who will support and help others.

Having reviewed and classified the obstacles and limitations, the health worker or team should look again at the objectives and change or adapt them if necessary, possibly by arranging specific activities to remove or reduce some of the obstacles; for instance, a survey to obtain missing information, training to produce skilled staff, etc.

The outcome of this exercise would be an analysis of obstacles and limitations and a revised list of objectives and targets.

Example: Some obstacles to antenatal care

Objectives and targets have been set and the health team must make sure that there are no obstacles to their achievement.

Consider the target set on page 292, "to provide 60% of pregnant women in the district with antenatal care during the current year". Obstacles to achieving this target are (in a given district):

— lack of transport for staff
— impassable mountain roads
— lack of interest among the women
— shortage of trained personnel.

Can these obstacles be overcome so that there is a good chance of meeting the target? A table is prepared to analyse the obstacles:

Objective	Obstacle or limitation	Analysis: obstacle can		Obstacle cannot be changed (in the short term)
		be removed	be modified	
To provide antenatal care to 60% of pregnant women	Impassable mountain roads		Use resident birth attendants	
	Shortage of midwives	Train and supervise traditional birth attendants	Changed function of midwives: to train, support and supervise traditional birth attendants	
	Women not interested	Particular care for women at risk		Education level of women
	Lack of official transport for staff		Use public transport	

Summary — Step 4

- **Ask the question "What is, or could be, preventing the achievement of the objectives?"**
- **Review limitations of resources — people, equipment, information, money and time.**
- **Review obstacles in the geographical, climatic, technical and social environment.**
- **Analyse obstacles/limitations to discover to what extent they can be removed or reduced.**
- **Revise objectives accordingly.**

Step 5: Scheduling the activities

Learning objectives

After studying Step 5 and doing Exercises 63 and 64 on pages 372–374, the health worker should be able to:

— **consider alternative strategies**

— **tabulate needed and available resources**

— **select the best strategy, taking account of obstacles and resources**

— **mobilize community resources**

— **detail activities**

— **write a plan.**

Once objectives and targets have been set and obstacles analysed, the health team and the community must plan how these objectives and targets may be achieved. There may be several different courses of action for achieving them.

A set of activities to meet objectives and targets is sometimes called a 'strategy', which means planning and using resources in ways that give the best chance of success.

Before planning activities in detail it is therefore necessary to:

— consider alternative ways of overcoming obstacles and achieving objectives
— balance resources and needs
— choose the best course of action

and then

— explain in detail the necessary activities, based on the chosen course of action.

Considering alternative courses of action

A valuable approach consists in getting people's ideas about simple ways of overcoming or reducing obstacles or limitations. Obstacles and limitations should first be discussed as individual problems and then as groups of related topics. Community representatives should be involved in all discussions.

When resources are limited, two general principles apply:

● The best use should be made of available resources before others are requested.

● Maximum use should be made of the most readily available resource before other resources are mobilized.

Different strategies rely more or less on one type of resource or another (or on combinations of resources), such as:

— infrastructure (e.g. buildings, communications)
— personnel (professionally qualified or auxiliary)
— equipment and supplies (either traditional or high-technology, but always appropriate)
— people (e.g. volunteers, village health committees, family members)
— capital expenditure or recurrent costs.

For instance, primary health care strategies are primarily people-oriented: they rely very little on complex infrastructure, make the best use of scarce trained manpower, rely on appropriate traditional technology, and do not cost more in capital or recurring expenses than the community can afford.

The general principle in designing alternative strategies for overcoming non-resource obstacles is to adapt to the physical environment (climate, terrain), and to choose methods that the community understands and accepts and that suit the country's administrative and political practices and the economic development of the area.

Thus, primary health care strategies will fit into the local situation by avoiding certain factors that are, or could become, obstacles to their implementation and by taking advantage of other factors for introducing acceptable changes in services.

ALTERNATIVE STRATEGIES HAVE BEEN CONSIDERED

Balancing resources and needs

To assist in deciding on a plan of action, it is helpful to draw up a list or table of resources required for different strategies, and a list of the various possibilities, noting whether each required resource is available or can be provided.

The review of resources should include the community's own resources — mainly people. It should also include buildings such as community meeting-houses where health activities could be carried out, materials such as wood for construction, transport such as boats, animals or the local bus service, and perhaps money. The possibility of better use of land and water for increased food production may be considered, e.g. vegetable plots or fish farms, as well as the more efficient and hygienic use of local water sources.

Through village leaders and designated representatives, the community should take an active part in this review. A plan should be drawn up, *within the limits of available resources,* even if this constraint means curtailing some activities at first. It is important to look at the priorities and consider how resources can be used for the maximum benefit of the whole population. Alternative ways of using resources, or the use of fewer resources, may need to be considered; for example, in some countries, using public transport may be an alternative to purchasing an expensive vehicle and paying for a driver, running costs, maintenance and repairs.

The advantage of planning in this way is that it ensures that some change takes place. Progress will be made towards achieving targets. Only when all available local resources have been put into use should requests for extra resources be made. Sometimes plans are made that rely too heavily on donations or on extra-governmental funds; if funds are not granted from these sources, or not sustained for a sufficiently long time, such plans will fail.

> **NEEDED RESOURCES HAVE BEEN REVIEWED**

Example: Alternative strategies for antenatal care to overcome limitations and obstacles

The following strategies might be considered for dealing with the shortage of trained midwives, transport difficulties and lack of interest among women in

302 ■ Part IV. Managing primary health care services

maternal and child health care:

1) *Mobilize* midwives by providing them with transport. This would help to increase women's interest, but would not solve the problem of impassable roads.

2) Find one or two women in each village who can be good *leaders* and who will encourage other women to become interested in, and use, the MCH services. However, this would not bring the services closer to the people or increase the acceptability or capacity of services.

3) Introduce the *risk approach* in the existing services, i.e. focus antenatal services and referrals on women at high risk. This would relieve pressure on staff, show the value of antenatal care, and thus raise interest among women. Lack of transport, however, would remain a handicap.

4) Improve the quantity and quality of services provided by *traditional birth attendants* (TBAs) in the villages, by introducing antenatal care into their routine work, through training and supervision by the health centre's midwife.

5) Use a combination of strategies 1, 2 and 3 (midwifery services, village leadership, risk approach).

6) Use a combination of strategies 2, 3 and 4 (village leadership, risk approach, TBAs).

The six alternative courses of action, or strategies, should be considered in joint meetings of health staff and community representatives. To choose the best way to overcome obstacles and limitations, each possible solution must be considered in relation to the resources it requires and those that are or could be made available.

Thus, the resources needed and available could be listed as in the table on p. 303.

In such a table, alternative strategies may be compared in terms of required and available resources, community acceptability and participation, and access to services. This makes selection of a strategy easier.

All members of the health team should take part in the review of resources and agree on the choice of course of action.

Choosing the best course of action

The choice of activities in any country, district or area depends on circumstances. In many cases, there is more than one choice. For example, TBAs could be trained and, meanwhile, a long-term plan for a future clinic could be started. The TBAs would deal with normal deliveries and the clinic would deal with referred complications.

Resources required (R) or available (A)

Type of resource	Alternative 1 R	Alternative 1 A	Alternative 2 R	Alternative 2 A	Alternative 3 R	Alternative 3 A	Alternative 4 R	Alternative 4 A	Alternative 5 (=1+2+3) R	Alternative 5 (=1+2+3) A	Alternative 6 (=2+3+4) R	Alternative 6 (=2+3+4) A
Skilled TBAs	—	✓	—	✓	—	✓	✓	✓	—	✓	✓	✓
Buildings	—	—	—	—	—	—	—	—	—	—	—	—
Transport	Heavy-duty jeep	—	—	—	—	—	—	—	Heavy-duty jeep	—	—	—
Educational materials	—	—	✓	—	✓	—	✓	—	✓	—	✓	—
Handbooks	—	✓	—	—	✓	✓	✓	✓	✓	✓	✓	✓
Supplies	—	—	—	✓	—	✓	✓	—	✓	✓	✓	✓
Roads	✓	Some not passable	✓	Some not passable	✓	Some not passable	—	—	✓	Some not passable	—	—
Capital cost	10 000		—		—		—		10 000		—	
Recurrent cost	2 000	✓	1 000	✓	1 000	✓	3 000	✓	4 000	✓	5 000	✓
Staff time (h): midwife	3 000	2 000	2 000	2 000	2 000	2 000	2 000	2 000	3 000	2 000	2 000	2 000
TBAs	—	—	—	—	—	—	40 000	40 000	—	—	40 000	40 000
Village women leaders	✓	✓	✓	✓	✓	✓	✓	✓	✓	✓	✓	✓
Population served	100%	60%	100%	60%	100% (at risk)	90% (at risk)	100%	70%	100% (at risk)	90%	100% (at risk)	90% (at risk)
Service available	Weekly in villages		Daily at health centre		Daily at health centre, monthly in villages		Daily in villages and at health centre		Weekly in villages, daily at health centre		Daily in villages and at health centre	

In introducing the design of alternative strategies, certain criteria were mentioned. These criteria may be applied in selecting the 'best' course of action:

● It should be the strategy that requires the least amount of scarce resources, but at the same time makes the maximum use of available resources.

● It should be the strategy that best suits the community environment, values and behaviour, i.e. introduces acceptable changes that encourage community participation in the proposed services.

● It should be the strategy that ensures the targeted quantity, quality and coverage of services required to achieve the objectives.

Selecting one of the alternative strategies reviewed

Alternative 6 from the example above is seen to be the best possible in the circumstances, for the following reasons:

● It does not depend heavily on costly transport.

● It mobilizes a valuable local resource, i.e. traditional birth attendants.

● It does not depend too much on the state of the roads.

● It does not require capital funding.

● It provides services at all times both in villages and at the health centre.

● It provides priority services to the women who most need them.

● It educates and motivates the female population.

What are the advantages of the chosen strategy?

● It will serve the greatest number of people.

● By training TBAs to give simple antenatal care and to discover women 'at risk', the health centre staff will have more time to spend on training and supervision and on dealing with complicated cases. Eventually, as more TBAs are trained and used, all pregnant women will receive antenatal care. Very little equipment is needed. The TBAs can 'learn by doing': even without equipment, they can learn to do many useful things.

● It is the strategy that the people want. They know the TBAs, who are always available to the people of the village.

A COURSE OF ACTION HAS BEEN CHOSEN

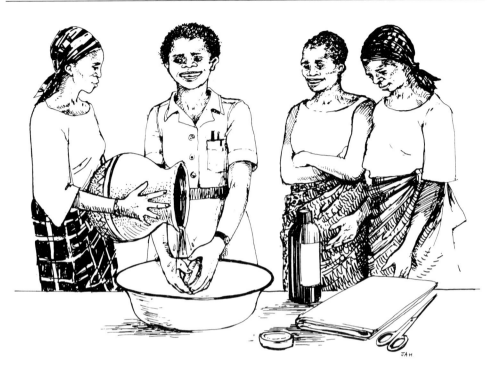

WHO 91319

Training traditional birth attendants

Example: District of Vosok

Nurse-midwife Shireen has decided that in her district the best choice of action is alternative 4, i.e. to train the traditional birth attendants in Sector A. This seems to be the only practicable way to reach the target of providing antenatal care for 60% of pregnant women within one year.

What will happen to the other 40%? They will continue to be served by untrained TBAs as before, but Nurse-midwife Shireen expects that all the TBAs will be trained within three years.

Shireen makes a list of everything a TBA could do to find and refer women at risk. A history of previous deliveries would indicate many possible risk cases. The TBA could also perform certain obstetric examinations without any equipment.

The midwife will spend more time training, supervising and supporting the TBA and less time doing the actual antenatal care herself. She will deal with all women referred to her by the TBA, and any woman she finds to be at risk during her supervisory visits.

Defining the chosen activities

Defining in detail the activities necessary for the chosen course of action again involves the health team and representatives of the community.

Thus, the activity "find traditional birth attendants" implies:

— a *survey* of those who practise traditional midwifery
— a *list* of TBAs
— *registration* of TBAs
— probably some *assessment* of the work-load, skill and performance of TBAs.

Similarly, the activity "train traditional birth attendants to give simple antenatal care" implies:

— *determining* the training needs of TBAs
— *motivating* TBAs to acquire new knowledge, skills and attitudes
— *preparing* learning materials for specific skills
— *training*
— *providing* TBAs with the necessary equipment and supplies to practise their new skills.

It may also imply:

— *assessing* the midwife's teaching and management skills
— *determining* the midwife's learning needs
— *training* the midwife
— *setting up* records and recording procedures
— *teaching* and *supervision*
    etc.

Implementation of the training programme may in turn involve *administrative* action such as obtaining approval for travel allowances, coordination of transport, etc.

As previously stated, an activity is something that is needed to pursue the course of action, something that can be clearly assigned to a person (TBA, midwife, supervisor, village head), something that can be performed (once or more often) within a certain period and for which some resources may be required (equipment, supplies, learning materials, records, allowances). Activities transform resources into results.

A schedule of activities shows the assignment of people's time and the desired product or result.

ACTIVITIES HAVE BEEN SCHEDULED

Writing an outline plan

A plan can be written in many ways. The order in which it is written depends on its main use or purpose. Sometimes governments or councils require plans in a specific form, especially when they are submitted to request funds or other resources.

In other cases, the order of headings used in writing a plan is less important. But the plan must always be written up under some system of headings, so that nothing is forgotten.

It is useful to write a brief summary of the whole plan and then to put details, such as lists of equipment, in an annex. Too much detail obscures the overview of a plan, but details are necessary so that the health worker who is responsible for managing the programme has full control of the implementation.

To ensure that money, people and equipment are available at the appropriate times, it is important to include a timetable — a list of detailed time-targets — as an annex to the plan.

In the example that follows, a plan is written under the seven guideline words: why, what, how, who, what, where, and when. It is followed by examples of detailed lists of time-targets, requirements and budget items for an antenatal and maternity care programme.

Example 1: An outline plan using the seven guideline words

Planning

Steps

1	*The information*	WHY are we doing this?
& 2	*The problem*	Explain the background, the problem to be solved, the reasons for the plan.

3 *Objective and targets*	*WHAT is to be done?* State what is expected to be achieved — both the main objective and the intermediate targets.
4 *Chosen strategy*	*HOW will it be done?*
& 5 *Activities*	Explain the strategy chosen, how it will overcome the obstacles, and the detailed activities necessary.

Implementing

| *Resources* | *WHO will do it?* |

People — How many are needed?
— What skills do they need?
— How will they be allocated?

WHAT things do we need?

Equipment — List equipment available
— List equipment to be ordered.

Money — Money available
(budget) — How is it to be used?
— How much more is needed?

| *Organization* | *WHERE will the work be done?* In which areas/villages/buildings will the plan be implemented? *WHEN will it be done?* Schedules of stages for activities to begin and end. |
| *Assignments* | Assign responsibility for activities. Decide on information to be collected for monitoring, and how it will be used. |

Example 2: Outline programme in maternal care

The problem	An isolated mountain community has no antenatal care and a high rate of maternal and neonatal deaths. The community is difficult to reach because of poor roads.
Objective	To give both antenatal and delivery care to about 60% of pregnant women within the next year.
Strategy and activities	The work is to be done by traditional birth attendants. The strategy is to train a nurse-midwife who will then train the TBAs. She will visit the village once a week for this purpose. Activities are detailed in Annex 1, below.

Resources	Nurse-midwife X has been chosen for a short course in the training of TBAs. Her job description is shown in Annex 2. The community will invite the TBAs to volunteer for training. Equipment lists and budget are shown in Annexes 3 and 4. [An analysis of resources such as that shown in the example on page 308 may also be included as a further annex.]
Organization	The training of TBAs will take place in the health centre and the village hall. The schedule for preliminary activities is shown in Annex 1.
Control	Each TBA will keep a simple record of her deliveries. These will be discussed each time the nurse-midwife visits the area. Problems can then be reviewed and advice given.

Annex 1: Detailed time-targets

	Sequence of activities	Time-targets
1. 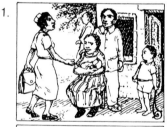	Visit to the community for discussions with people, to request donation of materials and clinic space, and to identify TBAs for training. Donated materials and space to be secured.	7 February 1 April
2. 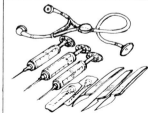	Equipment ordered Equipment received	2 April 5 May
3. 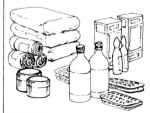	Medicine and material supplies ordered Supplies received	2 April 5 May

	Sequence of activities	Time-targets
	Education materials ordered Education materials received	2 April 5 May
	Funds requested for health worker's daily expenses Funds received	1 June 13 June
	Programme to be started	15 June

Annex 2: Job description for midwife in antenatal care work

A midwife is a health worker who has successfully followed the prescribed period of training, has passed the required examinations to obtain a diploma (or certificate) in midwifery, and is registered with the appropriate authority as a State Midwife.

The midwife is required to carry out the following tasks:

Promotional activities

To establish and maintain contact with TBAs, women of childbearing age, community leaders and other community development workers.

To use methods of demonstration, individual and group counselling, and learning and teaching, while working with TBAs, including:

— good personal hygiene
— good nutrition based on locally available foods
— organization of safe childbirth services
— education in methods of child-spacing.

Health care activities

To support the TBAs and carry out the following procedures and tasks for 'women at risk' referred by the TBAs for further care:

— confirming pregnancy
— weighing pregnant women
— checking blood pressure
— checking for anaemia, giving medication and advising on diet as indicated
— checking for vitamin deficiencies, giving medication and advising on diet as indicated
— examining for fluid retention
— testing urine
— determining pelvic measurements
— estimating approximate date of delivery
— identifying high-risk pregnancies
— explaining fetal development and maternal body changes
— demonstrating care of the newborn.

When needs are beyond her skill or when resources are not available, she will refer pregnant women at high risk to a higher level of care.

Information system

To register pregnant women.[1]
To register all activities carried out.
To register births and deaths related to the antenatal programme.
To prepare a monthly report of activities on the forms provided for the purpose, including training sessions for TBAs.
To forward the monthly report on the third day of the following month to the health centre.

Drugs and supplies

To report monthly on medicines and supplies used and the amount remaining.
To order, every six months, necessary replacements of medicines and supplies for the antenatal care programme.
To transport supplies from the health centre to the village.

---

[1] Registration may be done by a volunteer from the community, or by the TBA if she is literate, but the responsibility is ultimately the midwife's.

Training and experience

The health worker/midwife will have had training in learning and teaching methods, and experience in antenatal care under the direct supervision of a senior midwife.

Supervision

The midwife will perform her tasks under the supervision of the senior health worker at the health centre.

Annex 3: List of requirements for the maternal care programme

	Available	Required
People		
1 midwife or other health worker	✓	
Traditional birth attendants	✓	
(according to availability and population; maximum number in class = 8)		
Equipment for TBAs		
Non-expendable:		
Midwifery kits	✓	
Hand-washing basin	✓	
Waiting bench or mats		✓
Expendable:		
Soap	✓	
Referral cards		✓
(different colours for different problems if TBA is illiterate)		
Ferrous sulfate tablets	✓	
Flannelboard		✓
Equipment for midwife or health worker		
Non-expendable:		
Weighing scales	✓	
Haemoglobin test kit	✓	
Midwifery kit	✓	
Examination couch		✓
Test-tubes	✓	
Soap-dish	✓	
Hand-washing basin	✓	

	Available	Required
Equipment for midwife or health worker		
Non-expendable:		
Office chair	✓	
Desk	✓	
Waiting bench		✓
Expendable:		
Sheets	✓	
Cloth for examination screen	✓	
Towels	✓	
Soap	✓	
Referral cards	✓	
Maternal record cards	✓	
Register book	✓	
Medicines and laboratory supplies		
Ferrous sulfate tablets	✓	
Vitamin A capsules	✓	
Benedict's solution	✓	
Acetone-test powder	✓	
Educational materials		
Flannelboard	✓	
Nutrition models	✓	
'Growth of baby' models	✓	

Annex 4: Detailed budget for maternity programme

	Cost ($)
People	
Salary	
$40/day × 12 days/year × 1 health worker	480.00
Travel	
$0.40 per kilometre for 10 kilometres × 12 days/year × 1 health worker	48.00
Other allowances	
$10 per day × 12 days/year × 1 health worker (if training is required, the cost will be entered here)	120.00
Subtotal	648.00

		Cost ($)
Equipment		
Non-expendable:		
1 weighing scale at $70.00		70.00
1 haemoglobin test kit at $35.00		35.00
1 midwifery kit at $65.00		65.00
1 examination couch at $350.00		350.00
4 test-tubes at $0.45 each		1.80
1 hand-washing basin		5.00
1 soap-dish at $1.20		1.20
1 waiting bench at $55.00		55.00
	Subtotal	583.00
Expendable:		
4 towels at $2.00 each		8.00
8 soap bars at $0.30 each		2.40
50 referral cards at $20.00/100		10.00
100 maternal record cards at $20.00/100		20.00
1 register book at $5.00		5.00
	Subtotal	45.40
Medicine and laboratory supplies		
2 bottles ferrous sulfate tablets at $65/bottle		130.00
2 bottles vitamin A capsules (100 000) at $425/bottle)		850.00
1 litre Benedict's solution at $4.00/litre		4.00
1 g acetone-test powder at $5.00/g		5.00
	Subtotal	989.00
Educational materials		
1 flannelboard at $35.00		35.00
Food for nutrition demonstration (donated)		20.00
1 set 'Growth of baby' models at $30		30.00
	Subtotal	85.00
	Total programme cost	$2350.40
	Donated goods	20.00
	TOTAL BUDGET NEEDS	$2330.40

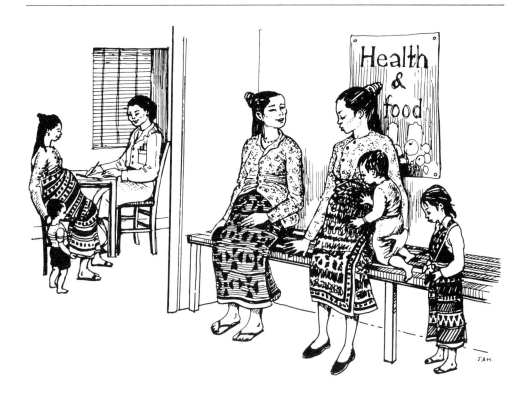

WHO 91320

Women 'at risk' are referred to the midwife or health centre

Summary — Step 5

- **Look at several ways of achieving the goal (alternative strategies).**
- **Make a table of resources needed and available for the different strategies. Always remember the resources within the community.**
- **Choose the most suitable alternative strategy.**
- **Make detailed activity schedules and budgets.**
- **Write an outline plan.**

CHAPTER 2
Implementing health activities

Introduction: The implementation function

Without implementation, plans remain theoretical. Management performs its implementation functions in order to put the principles discussed in Part I, Chapter 1, into practice.

The principles of division of labour and of delegation apply particularly to the management functions that deal with personal relationships. The principles of economy and substitution of resources apply to the management functions concerned with equipment, supplies and funds. The principle of management by exception, which applies primarily to information, affects the evaluation function and, through it, many implementation decisions. In implementation, management is concerned with achievement and performance.

Four main types of decision must be taken in implementation. The first type consists of all those that ensure that programme *activities* are executed as planned and services delivered as intended.

The second type concerns the deployment of *personnel* in the right numbers, at the right time and in the right place, to perform these activities.

The third deals with the mobilization and allocation of the physical and financial *resources* needed to perform the activities.

The fourth type of decision is concerned with the *information* needed, its processing, and its communication in support of the previous decisions and of evaluation.

Thus, these four types of implementation decision deal with:

— coordination of activities
— deployment of personnel
— allocation of resources
— processing of information.

Decisions about the coordination of activities

What is the exact nature of the day-to-day decisions concerned with the coordination of planned service, development and support activities? For any one activity to be implemented according to plan, management must make sure that all necessary preceding activities have been executed on time.

For instance:

> Retraining of TBAs is due next week. Necessary preceding activities were:
>
> — selection of candidate TBAs
> — preparation of learning materials
> — assignment of tutors
> — classroom arrangements.
>
> Management ensures that selected candidates have been informed, that the right number of workshop folders has been prepared, and that tutors and classrooms are available and ready.

The result of this check is either a decision to 'go ahead' (i.e. proceed with the retraining activity as scheduled) or a decision to modify the plan by altering the content, timing, location or other arrangements for the planned activity. Occasionally the decision may be to cancel the planned activity, to implement a contingency plan (an alternative plan that has been prepared to take account of unexpected circumstances), or to improvise (to decide on a different course of action without special preparation). Obviously such decisions depend on the decision-maker's information, terms of reference and operating rules. Typically, management reviews and modifies work schedules as a means of coordinating activities.

Decisions about the deployment of the workforce

The key management decisions that deal with deployment of the workforce to carry out the planned activities may be grouped under the following three broad headings:

— organizing
— directing
— supervising.

The following represent some decisions that relate to the *organization* function of management.

● For activities X, Y and Z, staff members A, B and C will perform the specified tasks — an *assignment decision*.
● For the proper coordination of activities X, Y and Z, staff meetings will be held at intervals to resolve issues of implementation that may arise — a *communication decision*.
● To assist staff to perform their assigned tasks, in-service training of midwives and TBAs will take place — a *staff-development decision*.

Job descriptions, standard operating procedures and duty rosters are the tools used by management in organizing work.

Examples of decisions pertaining to the *direction* of staff are:

● Staff assigned to activities X, Y and Z are *authorized* to undertake specified tasks — a *delegation decision*.

- In the performance of their duties, the staff assigned to activities X, Y and Z will be *answerable* to specified responsible officers — an *administrative control decision*.
- For the day-to-day direction of activities X, Y and Z, the activity leader will *exercise control* over specified sections and staff — a *decision about 'span of control'*.
- To ensure that activities X, Y and Z are successful, incentives will be provided to encourage participation and performance — a *promotional decision*.

Common *supervisory* decisions are concerned with:

- Applying agreed work standards and norms of performance, and specifying the procedures for the appraisal of staff performance.
- Identifying staff who need specific training for one or other aspect of their work.
- Supporting staff in the execution of their tasks.
- Resolving conflict.

A typical management instrument in this area is the supervision checklist.

It may be noted that organizing, directing and supervising are not entirely separate functions, and that some of the decisions mentioned under one heading above might well be placed under a different one. These types of decision belong to the *implementation* function of management, which has been described in more detail in Part II, Chapters 1 and 4.

Decisions about allocation of resources

At the implementation stage the type of decision concerned with the *allocation of resources* depends on the nature of the resource. Resources may be physical resources (such as equipment and supplies, including drugs), money, time and space, and information. Information, however, is a special type of resource, especially in the form of records, and is dealt with separately. The different types of decisions concern:

- *Monitoring and control* — All renewable resources need monitoring and control. This means watching availability, consumption and use (i.e. quantity), and quality (quality control), and, as appropriate, reordering, issuing, discarding, etc.

Time (a non-renewable resource) is similarly subject to monitoring and control decisions, so that it is used efficiently.

● *Logistics* Most physical resources also imply a logistic decision, i.e. the procurement, clearance, storage, forwarding (or dispatching), distribution, and replenishment of goods, both consumable (e.g. drugs) and non-consumable (e.g. vehicles).

● *Accounting* As a renewable resource, money is subject to accounting, a special form of monitoring and control, the purpose of which is to keep track of and compare receipts and expenditure, and to ensure that funds are expended only for the purposes for which they were allocated.

● *Organization* Some resources, like work-space and records, need organization. Organizational decisions are also generally necessary for physical resources (e.g. in regard to storage).

Decisions about the processing of information

Information is associated with decision-making in general, and with the coordination of activities in particular, as well as with the management of manpower and resources during implementation. The key decisions regarding information are as follows:

● *Why?* For each decision reviewed so far here, there is a specific information requirement.

● *What?* A decision must be made as to what constitutes the adequate quantity and quality of information. The criteria that information must satisfy in support of decision-making are: relevance, validity, reliability, timeliness and cheapness.

● *From where?* Once the nature of the information is identified, management must decide from which sources the particular information needed should be obtained or collected.

● *How?* The question of processing then arises, i.e. how information should be collated (put together), analysed, recorded, reported, etc. Processing may be undertaken in different places, by different people. Assigning these tasks is clearly a management decision.

● *To whom?*   Depending on the degree of specificity of the decision for which information is needed, it should be easy to decide to whom the information should be communicated.

The information that goes into a planned work (or activity) schedule often needs updating as implementation proceeds. An important management decision that has to be made from time to time concerns updating the schedule of activities (see pages 324–327).

The types of decision that concern information and its processing have been discussed in more detail in Part II, Chapter 5.

This completes the overview of the management functions in implementation. It should be clear to the reader that no one manager or decision-maker could cope with the whole of the function outlined above. Obviously the management function in implementation is a shared responsibility; who has which share must be clearly specified.

Summary

● **Implementation functions of management are concerned with day-to-day decisions about the timely execution of activities; with the organization, direction and supervision of personnel; with the mobilization, allocation, and monitoring and control of physical and financial resources; and with the processing and communication of the necessary information.**

● **These functions must be shared by the members of the health team.**

2.1 Coordinating the work of the health team

With the formulation of the plan, the most difficult part of the process is reached — how to implement the plan. Planning is designed to help implementation. The plan is a checklist and a guide; it is not something developed in isolation from existing activities.

A programme is a group or series of continuing and related activities designed to achieve a definite purpose or objective. It is a course of action designed to implement a plan or part of a plan. Stage by stage, the activities necessary to fulfil the plan are implemented so that the work is gradually completed. Changes take place and are integrated into existing programmes or become the beginning of new programmes.

For instance:

> A maternal and child health programme provides antenatal care to 50% of pregnant women. The objective of the plan is to extend this service over a period of time to all pregnant women. Implementing the plan means carrying out all the activities necessary for all pregnant women to receive care. The plan will then have achieved its objective, and antenatal care for all pregnant women will be an integral part of the maternal care programme.

As part of the management function the health worker:

1) Reviews the plan's objectives.
2) Reviews activities for each objective and target.
3) Checks the timetable. The timetable is essential for implementation; it states exactly when an activity must begin and end.
4) Verifies assignment of responsibilities to staff according to the activity schedules and job descriptions.
5) Discusses the implementation with representatives of the community, health service staff and workers in other sectors, where appropriate. The community decides how it can participate.
6) Checks the above items 1 to 5 against the seven guideline words: *why, who, when, what, which, where* and *how*.

To coordinate the work of the health team the health worker-in-charge must:

— coordinate the functions of the members of the health team
— coordinate the activities
— communicate the decisions.

Coordinating the functions of the health team

The need to coordinate the functions of the people working in a programme has been discussed briefly in Part II, Chapter 3.

Coordination is easier if there is a clear *organizational chart*, describing the relationships of the members of the service to one another.

Example

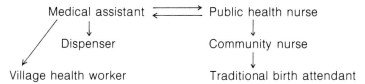

Organizational structure determines how communication takes place between the different levels of a system for the purpose of coordinating a programme and the activities of a health team. It specifies:

— who instructs others in what they are to do at each level of the organization
— to whom each person reports on progress or problems.

Often there is a three-level direct-line relationship in an organizational structure, as the following example illustrates.

Example

Midwife Aktar works in Sector A. She is supervised by the health area 'manager', Nurse-midwife Shireen. Midwife Aktar sends monthly reports to the health centre.

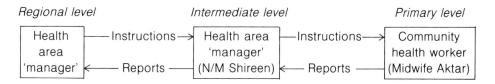

Clear *job descriptions* help people to work together harmoniously. (See Part II, Chapter 3.) The relations between staff members are strengthened if they all have clear individual job descriptions and know to whom they are accountable for their actions. However, the job description must be seen as a guide. It must not be used as an excuse for failing to help others who may, at times, have a heavier work-load, or for refusing to take part in activities not included in the description.

Coordinating the activities

It is not enough to list the activities necessary to the plan: the list must be put into a schedule or timetable. The schedule must state the time for beginning and completing each activity and who is responsible for seeing that it is completed on time.

To make a schedule, the programme must be reviewed as follows:

What should be done?   *Programme content*, e.g. content of the antenatal programme.

How it should be done?   *Procedures*—technical, administrative, managerial, etc.

Who should do it?   *People* responsible for the different tasks — health workers, administrative staff, community workers, etc.

When it should be done?   *Time-targets* to be followed.

How much it costs?   *Budget.*

Scheduling is the last step in planning (see Part IV, Chapter 1, page 299); the principles of planning have already been discussed (also in Part IV, Chapter 1, page 267). Implementation often calls for the revision or updating of planned schedules.

Revising and updating activity schedules

Work plans and activity schedules may need frequent revision and adjustment. Some activities may be completed ahead of schedule and others may be delayed. Unforeseen obstacles may arise to the achievement of targets or objectives; gaps appear between what was planned and what takes place. Keeping activity schedules up to date is therefore an important function of management, related to monitoring and control.

It has been pointed out that some activities, such as many service activities, are continuous, i.e. they occur all the time or at least at some point every day. Other activities, such as staff meetings and staff training, are sporadic, i.e. they occur from time to time. Others are one-time activities, i.e. they occur only once; examples are purchasing a vehicle or designing a records system. In preparing or reviewing a schedule of activities, as well as the assignment of staff, these differences must be kept in mind.

It is a common feature of all activities that they *produce* something — a product or service, for instance. Certain products are essential, or critical, to the smooth operation of a programme or service and to the achievement of the stated objectives. For instance, no training can take place without students and learning materials. The activities that result in these products are therefore essential and must be provided and coordinated and indicated in the activity schedule concerned with the training course.

In the strategy mentioned on page 302, "TBAs trained in the risk approach", the trained TBA is such a critical product. If the health-centre midwife is responsible for providing this training, she must be completely familiar with the risk approach and have prepared (or obtained) the necessary learning materials — another critical product. As course organizer, she must know of TBAs in the community and be in a position to select several for the course and thus make a list of candidates. This list — and some evidence of the TBAs' present competence and learning needs — is therefore a third critical product for the implementation of the strategy.

To produce a list of TBAs' training needs, in preparation for the training course, the essential or prerequisite activities might include:

1) a census of the women of childbearing age
2) a survey of prevalent delivery practices
3) the registration of practising TBAs
4) an assessment of the performance of the TBAs
5) selection of the TBAs to be trained
6) systematic derivation from the above 'products' 1 to 5 of the learning needs, i.e. the specific skills the TBAs need to acquire, and the methods by which they will acquire these skills.

Similarly, to produce the necessary learning materials, the essential activities might include:

— assessing the midwife-trainer's skill in the risk approach and in preparing educational materials
— determining her learning needs, i.e. the skills she lacks or needs to improve
— her actual training
— the provision of materials and equipment, and the facilities needed for producing and organizing them for the TBAs' learning purposes.

Rescheduling must take place if the sequence is blocked or has to be broken — for instance, if the midwife is transferred to a new posting just as she has completed her own training, and another midwife must replace her. The sequence must then be interrupted and can be resumed only after the new midwife arrives and is trained, if necessary, to prepare the educational materials. In any case, the training courses may have to be postponed. The new scheduling will depend on when the learning materials are available and this in turn may depend on another set of activities — administrative activities — leading to the appointment of a new midwife. These administrative activities (advertising the post, screening the candidates, selecting and transferring the new midwife) will delay the course, perhaps by several months, and therefore the activities ending with the training course must be rescheduled.

At the same time as the midwife is being trained to conduct the TBA course and the learning materials are being prepared, other activities must be carried out, such as:

— selecting the villages or sectors in which particular aspects of TBA training are to take place
— determining the sequence in which training in different villages or sectors is to take place (if different groups of TBAs are to be trained separately)
— consulting with the community leaders concerned
— arranging the necessary support activities.

When these activities have been completed, the activities leading to "TBAs trained in the risk approach" may be sequenced village after village or sector after sector over a period of, say, three to six months.

Such rescheduling of activities is a management task and implies monitoring and control — the subject of the next chapter.

Coordination does not end with rescheduling: decisions must be communicated to the interested parties.

Communicating the decisions

What decisions result from using the coordination instruments reviewed above?

Obviously — rescheduling decisions affecting one or more activities.
Consequently — reassignment decisions, shifting staff time from one or more tasks to other tasks or activities.
This entails — reallocation to other activities or functions of resources freed by rescheduling.

And possibly — revision of job descriptions, duty rosters and work timetable.

Occasionally — revision of objectives and targets.

However well the planned activities are scheduled and the organizational
chart and job descriptions are written, coordination will not succeed until
decisions and work directives are communicated and understood by all
members of the team.

An organizational chart may be placed on the wall of the health centre
and discussed with the members. Each health worker should have an
individual job description in writing.

The activities schedule should be reviewed and discussed with the health
team and with the community to determine whether the time-targets are
feasible and realistic.

Summary

To coordinate work effectively, the health worker must:

- **clarify jobs and relationships so that people work together harmoniously**
- **reschedule activities as needed**
- **communicate decisions to all concerned with the work.**

2.2 Monitoring and redirecting work (control)

Many health activities take place at the same time, and the health team
needs certain 'tools' to watch, or monitor, the work. The purposes of
monitoring are as follows:

- *Monitoring of inputs* ensures that:
    - work progresses according to schedule
    - staff are available (in accordance with assignments)
    - resource consumption and costs are within planned limits
    - the required information is available
    - community groups or individuals participate as expected.

- *Monitoring of process* ensures that:
  - the expected functions, activities and tasks are performed in accordance with set norms
  - work standards are met
  - meetings are held as needed
  - communications take place as necessary.

- *Monitoring of outputs* ensures that
  - products meet specifications
  - services are delivered as planned
  - training results in new skills or higher levels of skill
  - decisions are timely and appropriate
  - records are reliable and reports are issued
  - conflicts are resolved
  - the community is satisfied.

Obviously monitoring does not achieve all of this by itself. Where there are deficiencies, control decisions must follow the observations, and such decisions often involve more complicated processes (described in Chapter 3).

To summarize the above statements, it may be said that monitoring and control are concerned with:

- work progress
- staff performance
- service achievement.

Monitoring provides the information, and matches it with set norms or standards; control follows recognition or discovery of deficiencies.

Maintaining work standards

A health worker must be able to:

- use checklists to observe performance and recognize deficiencies in procedures, standards and output
- trace the causes of work deficiencies (i.e. the personal, technical, administrative or organizational reasons for standards not being achieved).

The usefulness of a checklist has been discussed in other chapters. A checklist is like a set of criteria; health workers can prepare checklists to assist in monitoring their own activities. A checklist is also a record or a reminder of what is happening, and can be used as a basis for planning future activities and for following up progress.

There are many causes of work deficiencies. Work is assessed periodically to detect such deficiencies and their causes, and to remedy them before they become too serious. Sometimes the cause may be a technical fault in a piece of equipment, but it may be a fault of organization, such as failure to train a rural health worker for certain tasks in order to reduce the demands on an overworked nurse.

The fault may lie with the staff or with the administration. For example, reports may arrive at the health centre late or not at all; this, in turn, may be because previous reports were not acknowledged or followed up. Acknowledging reports from the village, and letting it be known that the contents are of interest and useful, will encourage village health workers to send reports in, and to do so on time.

Sometimes a work deficiency can be remedied by retraining (see Part II, Chapter 3).

A supervisor who is monitoring is continually checking on health service activities, noting shortcomings that need attention, and asking the question, "Is the programme or service operating as intended?".

For instance:

>Do the health units receive adequate drug supplies?
>Are the leprosy clinics being held regularly?
>Do the midwives complete the MCH cards correctly?
>Is the referral system being used as intended?

Methods of monitoring

Methods of monitoring equipment and resources are described in Part III. A supervisor monitors work by:

— continually observing work progress, staff performance and service achievements
— checking supplies against inventories and stock-lists
— examining records
— discussing progress and difficulties with staff and with the community.

Information obtained from monitoring is used to identify day-to-day problems as well as for yearly planning of the health work for the area. It is essential to be aware of the significance of the information and to be confident of its accuracy. Records must be reviewed at regular intervals and information must be verified. The following are four examples of the analysis and verification of information.

Example 1

In the monthly checking of the stock ledger and inventory it is noticed that nearly all of the two months' supply of oral rehydration mixture has been used in the first month.

● A problem has been found during a regular record review.

Is the information correct or was there an error in recording the amounts?

The supervisor checks the monthly reports to find out whether the information on the amount of mixture used corresponds with the number of people who were treated for diarrhoea, and finds that more people than usual received this treatment.

● Information has been verified by checking with another record.

Example 2

A review of monthly reports shows that the number of new attendances at antenatal clinics is falling each month. According to the information available about women of childbearing age, the number of pregnant women receiving antenatal care should be increasing.

● A problem has been found during a regular report review.

The information may also be verified in other ways, such as talking with the villagers or village leaders.

To be sure that the reports are accurate, the supervisor talks with the health worker who wrote the monthly report, and finds that the information is correct.

● Information is verified by talking to the village health worker and villagers.

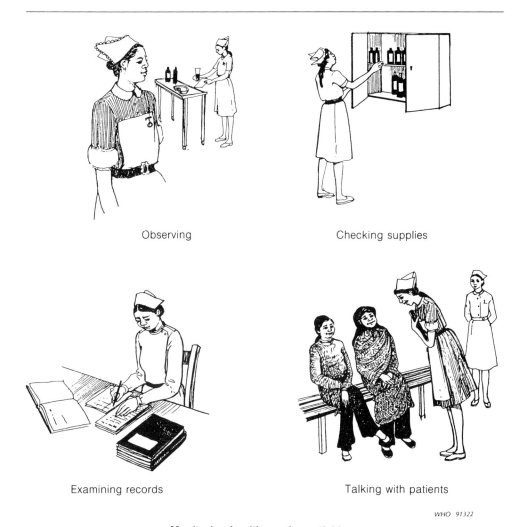

Observing

Checking supplies

Examining records

Talking with patients

WHO 91322

Monitoring health service activities

Example 3: Monitoring progress towards target

The objective is: "to give antenatal care to 60% of the pregnant women in Sector A in one year".

Is the objective being reached? Management tools that measure quantity or output of work will help in answering this question.

Information from the health workers, such as the monthly report of new pregnancies, will reveal how many different pregnant women were given care during a month. Adding the totals of new cases (not revisits) together month by month (cumulative total) will show the exact number of pregnant women who have received care to date. This number can be compared with the target of 60%, to see whether the work is progressing as expected.

The supervisor has received monthly reports for the past six months from the health worker in Sector A. Cumulative totals made each month for the antenatal programme are as follows:

Month	Number of pregnant women receiving antenatal care (new patients)	Cumulative totals
January	3	3
February	5	8 (5+3)
March	7	15 (8+7)
April	6	21 (15+6)
May	8	29 (21+8)
June	10	39 (29+10)

The target set for the programme was that 60% of expectant mothers were to receive antenatal care. The expected number of deliveries for the year was 138 and the target of 60% is 77. The cumulative total number of women under care to date is 39, which shows that the programme has reached half the target at the end of six months. The target for the year is therefore likely to be met.

If work progress is not up to norm, the reason must be identified. The following example shows some of the questions that must be asked and the corresponding management tools that must be used to help find out why targets are not being met.

Example 4: Investigation of antenatal programmes

Questions	Management tools
Is the work planned efficiently?	Supervisory checklist.
Has the health worker established good community relationships?	Talk with the people.
Are the TBAs participating well in the training?	Supervisory visit with midwife and TBAs.
Do TBAs provide antenatal care to pregnant women at home?	Reports from midwife.
Do TBAs assist with group antenatal sessions in the health centre?	Supervisory visit.
Are the necessary supplies available?	Inventory of stocks.

Questions	Management tools
Is the programme wanted and accepted by the people?	Talking with the people and examining pregnant women.
Is early action being taken to fulfil needs identified in the supervisory visits?	Supervisory checklist indicating months of visits and action taken.
Do you feel the action chosen was the best one? Are there problems that were not revealed during the planning period?	Talking with the health worker and the people.
Is there a coordination problem?	List of intermediate activities.
Were the activities planned for the programme adequate?	Programme plan (stating procedures, time elements, etc.).

Redirecting activities (control decisions)

When it is found that targets are not being met, it is often necessary to redirect the programme and sometimes to modify the goals.

Example

Monitoring shows that antenatal care targets in Health Sector A are not being met. The reason for this is that some TBAs are hostile to the training programme. They do not give antenatal care. The women they will deliver do not wish to attend the group clinic.

The nurse-midwife thinks that this problem can be overcome through a group approach. First, she discusses the problem with the midwife; together, she and the midwife then see community leaders. Finally they talk with all the TBAs, especially those who have not yet taken part in the training and antenatal programmes.

Meanwhile the midwife spends an extra day each month in Health Sector A, devoting more time to work with the TBAs and among the women who will be delivered by the TBAs.

Time is thus an important element. The midwife must adjust her timetable and activities. The nurse-midwife must also adjust her timetable for a month or two to permit her to spend more time in visiting Health Sector A, supporting the midwife and helping her consolidate the antenatal programme. This will mean delegating certain tasks to another member of the health centre staff. Since this programme will, if successful, be a model for other villages in the area, the nurse-midwife feels that the time spent with the midwife is worth while.

Summary

- **Monitoring means watching the progress, achievements and standards of work of a programme.**
- **Monitoring can be done by every staff member, with the help of a checklist, by means of interviews and discussions, and by studying records and reports.**
- **Monitoring may result in a programme being redirected.**

2.3 Supervision in action

Various styles of supervision were discussed in Part II, Chapter 2. Whichever style is adopted, the *activities* of supervision remain similar. This chapter discusses some of these supervisory activities in relation to:

- *Objectives.* Supervision is one way to:
  — make sure that objectives correspond to needs
  — discuss, explain, justify, and obtain the commitment of health workers to the objectives of the programme
  — make sure that there are no divergences between the objectives of management (e.g. standards of performance), the objectives of the staff and the objectives of the users
  — seek solutions to any conflict that arises between management, staff and users regarding the programme objectives.

- *Performance.* Supervision is the way to:
  — observe how the tasks entrusted to different categories of worker are carried out, and under what conditions
  — analyse the factors that result in satisfactory performance and the obstacles to satisfactory performance (knowledge and attitudes of workers, environment, resources)
  — determine, with the health workers, the causes of difficulties.

- *Staff motivation.* Supervision is one way to:
  — obtain a clear picture of health workers' fundamental needs (especially the need to 'belong', the need for respect, and the need for a sense of achievement)
  — help staff develop the necessary maturity to accept responsibility, especially by discovering and discussing work-related factors that enhance or diminish motivation
  — discover shortcomings in staff skills in communication, problem-solving, and resolution of conflict
  — adapt the leadership style of supervisors to staff's expectations.

- *Staff competence.* Supervision is one way to:
  — determine staff needs for information on the community, on health problems, on programme goals, and on standards to be attained
  — determine the skills required by staff for care, management, etc.
  — decide jointly on appropriate learning methods for acquiring or improving these skills
  — set up a programme of continuing education.

- *Resources.* Supervision is one way to:
  — identify particular needs for logistic or financial support.

Supervision, therefore, concentrates on people and sets out to improve performance. It is justified mainly by the fact that it gives the supervisor the opportunity not only to provide guidance, advice and help, but also to learn.

Making a supervisory schedule

Either one health worker or several may be assigned to different villages in a health area. In either case a supervisory plan must be made for each year. The frequency of supervisory visits will depend on the local situation, the state and stage of the programme, and the availability of transport and personnel.

Planning the schedule for supervisory visits includes:

— deciding how often supervisory visits are needed
— listing all programmes
— determining the need for supervision (checklist)
— noting the aspects of health care where special assistance is required (checklist).

Step 1: Listing the health activities or programmes where supervision is most needed

A listing such as that shown below enables a supervisor to note reasons for making more frequent visits, and thus to plan for them in order to maintain the control needed to reach programme goals.

Programme	Extra needs for control	Health areas		
		A	**B**	**C**
1) Antenatal	New programme: one visit a month for six months from July	✓		
2) Nutrition	Coordination with other agency workers: one visit a month for six months from July	✓		
3) Immunization	Reorganized activity: visits in January and June	✓	✓	✓
4) Water supply	New health worker: one visit a month		✓	

Step 2: Reviewing other timetables

The next step in scheduling is to arrange a timetable for the supervisory visits. Two things are needed for this:

- The plan made for the year. This shows the definite dates allotted to fixed events. (Refer to Part III, Chapter 4, Section 4.6.)

- The health unit timetable or schedule. This shows the days of the week allotted to regular activities. (Refer to Part III, Chapter 4, Section 4.2.)

Step 3: Making a yearly schedule for supervisory visits

The yearly schedule for supervisory visits is then planned as shown below, taking into account:

— minimum needs for supervisory visits
— programme needs for more frequent supervisory visits
— fixed dates in the annual plan
— fixed activities that happen regularly each week.

Month	Area A	Programme number	Area B	Programme number	Area C	Programme number
Jan.	1st Mon.	3	2nd Mon.	3	3rd Mon.	3
Feb.			2nd Mon.	4		
Mar.	1st Mon.	all	2nd Mon.	4	3rd Mon.	all
Apr.			2nd Mon.	4		
May	1st Mon.	all	2nd Mon.	4	3rd Mon.	all
Jun.	1st Mon.	3	2nd Mon.	3	3rd Mon.	3
Jul.	1st Mon.	1+2				
Aug.	1st Mon.	1+2	2nd Mon.	all	3rd Mon.	all
Sep.	1st Mon.	1+2				
Oct.	1st Mon.	1+2	2nd Mon.	all	3rd Mon.	all
Nov.	1st Mon.	1+2				
Dec.	1st Mon.	1+2	2nd Mon.	all	3rd Mon.	all

The visits outside the health centre are planned so as to keep the fourth week of each month free for completing required monthly reports.

After the supervision schedule has been made, health workers in the areas to be visited should be told the dates of the visits so that they will be available. The village leaders should also be informed, as they, or the people, may wish to talk with the visiting health worker.

When the yearly schedule for supervisory visits has been prepared, arrangements must be made for transport to be available on the days of visits to the villages.

Preparation for supervisory visit

Before making a supervisory visit the health worker should review records with regard to, for example:

— local targets
— the health worker's activities in the programme to be observed
— progress to date of the programme in relation to set targets
— problems in implementing the programme
— supplies needed.

Example

In making the August work-plan, the supervisor notes that a visit is scheduled to Health Sector A because extra supervisory help is needed for the new programme of antenatal care. To prepare for the visit the following checks are made:

- The health worker's *job description* is reviewed.
- The *monthly report* from the health worker in Sector A is reviewed to determine the number of pregnant women who have received care. This number is checked against the target set for the antenatal programme, so that the progress of the programme to date may be assessed.
- *Supervisory checklists* for Sector A from the previous supervisory visit are checked to see whether some items must be followed up, whether any on-the-job training is needed, and whether any other problems have been noted.
- The *inventory of medicines and supplies* is checked to see whether Sector A needs supplies that the supervisor could take.

A small supervision notebook helps in planning visits. The health worker can note in it information from records kept at the health centre, as well as a list of topics to be discussed during the visit. The notebook is an informal record, and notes can be made in any way that the health worker finds easy and most useful.

Example

The health manager has checked records in order to plan a supervisory visit to the health worker in Sector A, and has written in the notebook:

Sector A

Visit planned for second Monday in June. (Check available transport during 1st week June.) Health worker began work 1 December.

1) Are targets being met?
2) Do close check of technical competence in antenatal care.
3) Take supplies for 2 months.
4) Talk with people in the village to assess their health needs, and their attitudes towards the health worker.
5) Talk with midwife.

Conducting a supervisory visit

The most difficult part of supervision comes last, i.e. conducting the supervisory visit. Supervisors must always remember that *supervision is a helping process.*

Example

> The health worker/supervisor takes the supervisory checklist, notebook and supplies, and travels to Sector A to make a scheduled supervisory visit. The first part of the visit is planned to be a check of the records to verify the monthly report information. However, the health worker at the village health centre, as often happens, wants to discuss personal problems first. It is important to listen to the health worker and to try to discover the source of the problem.
>
> "I have too much to do" he complains. Does he have too much to do, or is this a problem of time-management? More information is needed.

The worker's records can be reviewed with him to assess the amount of work being done. Travel conditions, scheduling of work, and geographical conditions that might make travel time longer than necessary would then be discussed.

It would be good supervisory practice to suggest that the health worker keep a simple timetable of his activities. (Refer to Part III, Chapter 4, Managing time.) The results could be discussed during the next month's supervisory visit and better ways of using time suggested.

A poor supervisory response to this health worker's problem would be to say "Work faster", and then to continue with the routine activities of the supervisory visit. This could possibly result in the loss of a good worker because of lack of understanding and failure to listen and motivate.

Routine supervisory activities in Sector A, in accordance with the supervisory plan, would include:

- Looking at records to see whether they are well kept and whether they agree with monthly report information. ("Are targets being met?" had been noted in the supervisory notebook.)
- Observing how the health worker performs the activities listed in the job description, such as cleaning equipment and storing supplies, teaching people about health, and caring for the sick and injured.
- Talking with the village leader and other people. Do they understand and want the programmes that are being implemented? Do they feel that they need other help? They should be encouraged to talk about their needs as they see them and about how they feel that these needs might be met.

- Discussing with the health worker, at the end of the visit, what has been found: good points (health centre is clean, supplies are safely stored) as well as the need for improvement (wash hands before and after examining or treating sick people, tell them what to do to keep well) and how improvements might be made.

- Reminding the health worker of the date of the next supervisory visit to the area.

All the observations made should be noted on the supervisory checklist or in the notebook for follow-up, as needed.

On returning to the health centre the supervisor should arrange for follow-up of the noted items, so that information or solutions to problems may be found before the next planned visit.

Summary

The purpose of supervision is to help the health worker:
- **plan a schedule of visits for a year ahead**
- **keep a notebook for supervisory visits**
- **prepare the visit carefully beforehand**
- **use a supervisory checklist.**

CHAPTER 3
Evaluating health activities

Learning objectives

After studying this chapter and doing Exercises 70–73 on pages 379–388, the health worker should be able to evaluate:

— the achievements of a health team in services delivered and their impact in reducing the priority health problems of the community

— the progress of a health team's work

— the performance of the individual members of a health team

— the efficient use of the health team's resources

— the management of the health team.

Introduction: The evaluation function

As has been noted in Part I, evaluation is an essential part of management by objectives and learning from experience. Evaluation is also related to the principle of management by exception.

'To evaluate' is simply defined as *to judge the value of*. The term is often used incorrectly in the sense of 'to examine' or 'to measure' or 'to assess'. However, evaluation *depends* on examination or measurement or assessment, which must be carried out to obtain the information that will allow an evaluation to be made. Generally, the term 'evaluation' is used to include the whole process of examination or measurement and the ultimate judgement of value.

In this context, the term 'assessment', sometimes used as a synonym for evaluation, is normally used in relation to the observation of performance of students as they demonstrate clinical skills or competence in carrying out a health care activity or of health workers as they undertake a health care task.

Assessment of performance of staff is an essential part of evaluation of a health programme and is a direct means of measuring quality of health care.

The term 'appraisal' is normally used instead of 'evaluation' in relation to a supervisor's annual review of performance of individual health care staff.

The purpose of management (improving achievement and performance) and the nature of management decisions were discussed in Part I. Management decisions concerned with evaluation are those that deal with the health team's:

— effectiveness, or achievement of results
— performance of activities
— efficiency, or economic use of resources.

As evaluation is concerned in the first instance with *effectiveness*, or the achievement of results, the following questions are asked first:

● Are the results as intended?
● Are the results of value?

When the answer to both questions is 'yes', the most likely decision will be to carry on as planned. If the answer to either question is 'no', the ensuing decision will usually be to revise the objectives or the activities or both.

With regard to *performance*, the evaluator asks the following questions:

● Are the results as good as they could be?
● If not, why not?

When the results are as good as they could be, the decision will usually be to make no change. When results are less good than expected, however, the likely decision will be to change the design of activities or the use of staff or of other resources.

Finally, with regard to *efficiency*, the evaluator asks the questions:

● Could the same results have been achieved more cheaply?
● If so, by substituting what resources for those that were used?

If the results could have been achieved more cheaply, the ensuing decision would be to use resources more economically. This kind of typical 'control' decision might be taken, for instance, in preparing yearly operating budgets.

Before going on to a review of management functions in evaluation, it is worth emphasizing that evaluation can be undertaken at different times and in various ways, but that it follows certain general principles.

The general approach in evaluation is as follows:

— *measurement* of observed achievement
— *comparison* with previously stated norms[1], standards[2] or intended results
— *judgement* of the extent to which certain values are satisfied
— *analysis* of causes of failure
— *decision* (feedback).

For instance:

> According to its records, a health team has achieved an 80% coverage with postnatal visits in its health area. The target it had set itself was 75% coverage. Achievement therefore appears to be more than satisfactory. However, by looking at the distribution of the women who were visited, it appears that none belongs to any of three distant villages. This does not satisfy the community's demand for 'equal access to services'. A decision is therefore required.

This example illustrates an important difficulty in evaluating effectiveness. In the example, is effectiveness best measured as coverage, equal access to services, or both? Is the health team more successful if it exceeds its coverage target by concentrating its efforts on nearby villages than if it provides services equally to all the villages at the cost of lower coverage? Effectiveness is not a simple matter of success or failure.

In practice, a health team tries to meet the many and varied *needs* of the community and to satisfy its more pressing *demands*. It also has to pay attention to problems that have national priority, and therefore sets itself

---

[1] Norm: standard quantity to be produced or amount of work to be done.
[2] Standard: measure by which accuracy or quality is judged.

operational targets in a variety of programme areas (such as nutrition, water supply, communicable diseases, family health), as well as *time-frames* for their achievement. Effectiveness is about all of these aspects of the team's functions, and its evaluation should be concerned with all of them, provided that it is possible to obtain, from records or by measurement or assessment at reasonable cost and with reasonable effort, the necessary valid and relevant information.

The means of measuring effectiveness must therefore be carefully selected. Before the measurement of effectiveness for purposes of programme evaluation is begun, the following questions should be asked:

● What planning or implementation decisions will be affected by the findings?

● How will the findings be used in making those decisions?

● How, and to what extent, will implementation of the decisions improve effectiveness?

For instance:

> After the evaluation of the effectiveness of the health team in the above example, the following implementation decisions must be made:
>
> ● Ought the team to provide services to the three distant villages? If so, when? What proportion of the staff and resources should be reallocated for the purpose?
>
> ● Where could services in other villages be reduced and how could resources thus saved be used for the villages not yet covered? Information on the postnatal coverage of women in each village will show this.
>
> ● Should, say, 10% of staff time and other resources be transferred to the three distant villages? This would probably not reduce coverage to less than 75% in any of the other villages, but would raise coverage from 0 to 50% in the three distant ones, which would be a significant improvement in effectiveness.

From this example it can be concluded that 'coverage' and 'distribution' are suitable aspects of effectiveness to measure since they point to necessary implementation decisions, contribute to making such decisions, and support the decisions. However, there are other difficulties with evaluation.

For instance:

> A health team evaluates its effectiveness in providing clean water to
> the households in an area where the ratio of pumps to households
> was 1 to 45. The target was one pump to every 20 households. At the
> midpoint of the plan period the ratio is only one pump to every 40
> households. It seems that the team is failing to achieve the target.

The pump:households ratio is a valid but insufficient measure of the
team's effectiveness; it tells nothing about the possible cause of failure. To
learn from experience (which is one of the principal purposes of evaluation) something more must be done. It is essential to analyse what factors
are preventing successful implementation.

This implies looking at the entire chain of events that would normally
have resulted in success, and discovering what are the obstacles and
limitations that are preventing success, as well as the positive factors that
would lead to success if the team were to take them into account. In the
above example such analysis might include:

— estimating the community's demand for water
— examining community acceptance of the type of pump proposed
— finding out whether the community can pay for maintenance of the
  water supply system
— checking whether all the required parts are available in stock
— testing the drilling rig
— appraising the technical ability of those who prepared the detailed
  plans for the project
— finding out whether the rural water scheme is assured of adequate
  funds for reaching the target and maintaining the service.

This is a continuation of the evaluation, but in depth. Although evaluation may be concerned primarily with effectiveness, it will often reveal
inefficiency, or uneconomical use of scarce resources, as a cause of failure
to reach a target.

Sometimes the evaluation in depth can turn towards management itself,
asking the question "How efficient is the management?". This self-evaluation of management is usually referred to as *management audit*.

Obviously management needs information to be able to discuss seriously
such points as those raised in the example above. In Chapter 2, on
implementation, reference was made to the monitoring function of management as the mechanism for getting the right kind of information, where

and when it is needed, for evaluation purposes as well as for more immediate control purposes. In this sense, monitoring is part of the evaluation function of management.

Finally, *feedback* is necessary for learning from experience. When a health team undertakes an evaluation, with all members contributing, the feedback is immediate, in as much as every staff member learns from the discussion. However, evaluation findings and their interpretation must also be communicated to decision-makers at other levels, especially if their participation in improving the situation is expected. Feedback may be made available to the community, to its representatives and leaders, and to higher levels of administration.

Evaluation, particularly when it requires an analysis of causes of under-achievement, is the best way to ensure that management focuses attention on what matters most: it helps in making *big decisions first.*

3.1 Evaluating achievement

To evaluate a programme for its effectiveness is to judge the value of results achieved by the health team. It necessitates measuring the extent to which people get the services that were planned to meet their needs, and assessing how much they benefited from the services. The information thus obtained is used to improve the quantity, quality, accessibility, efficiency, etc. of services.

Two broad questions must be asked:

● Are the results those that were intended?
● Are they of value?

The general approach to evaluation (in this case, for effectiveness) consists of the following five steps:

— deciding what aspects of the programme are to be evaluated and how effectiveness is to be measured
— collecting the information needed to provide the evidence
— comparing the results with the targets or objectives
— judging whether and to what extent the targets and objectives have been met
— deciding whether to continue the programme unchanged, to change it, or to stop it.

Evaluation is often described as a continuous function, but in this chapter the evaluation of a single programme within a limited time period (e.g. in preparation for an annual report) is described. The evaluation is performed by health staff, who will be expected to collect and analyse the information needed as a basis for evaluation.

Decide what is to be evaluated and how effectiveness is to be measured

In principle, a plan should specify how each programme or activity it contains is to be evaluated and what will be accepted as evidence of satisfactory achievement. For instance, if the plan contains the following targets:

> "By the end of 1996, the incidence of neonatal tetanus in the 21 villages of Jaya District will be reduced to 1 per 1000 live births from the present (1992) incidence of 5 per 1000."

> and

> "By 1996 all the people in the district will have adequate access to preventive services (according to predetermined criteria of accessibility)."

it should provide also for the achievement of the targets to be measured by (a) the yearly incidence (i.e. number of cases) of neonatal tetanus per 1000 live births; (b) the rate at which the incidence falls from one year to another; and (c) the distribution of new cases among the 21 villages. The variables (a), (b) and (c) are therefore direct measures of the effectiveness of the programme.

Use of these measures during the plan period will show the progress being made in reducing the incidence of neonatal tetanus (i.e. monitoring). At the end of the period it will show whether the target has been achieved or what still remains to be done.

If interim targets have not been set during planning, those responsible for monitoring and evaluation should decide at the start of the programme what information must be collected to monitor and evaluate the programme. Ideally, baseline information (e.g. the yearly incidence and the distribution of neonatal tetanus before the target is set) should be obtained. However, it may be necessary to obtain or confirm this information at an early stage of the programme, and to change the target accordingly. Otherwise, it will be impossible to determine with certainty whether incidence is falling or whether any fall in incidence is a result of the programme.

Collect the necessary information

Evaluation requires that the information needed to monitor and evaluate progress is made continuously available throughout the plan period. Thus, for the purposes of this example, *every case* of neonatal tetanus must be reported to the monitoring and evaluation group, and reliable arrangements must be made to obtain the information at regular intervals (e.g. once a week, or on a fixed date each month).

There must be someone (e.g. a health volunteer) in each village who is responsible for recording and reporting the information, and a health-centre staff member (e.g. the public health nurse-midwife) who is responsible for collecting and processing the information at the end of every 3-month period.

Compare results with targets or objectives

At each monitoring point (e.g. every 3 months or at the end of each year), the information obtained must be compared with the targets set for that period or time and for each place. It is helpful if the information is laid out in a table that shows data by year (or other specified period) and place (e.g. each village in a district). The figures recorded in the table must be changed into rates (per cent or per thousand) to enable comparisons to be made, unless the targets themselves are expressed in figures rather than rates.

Continuing with the example of neonatal tetanus, three simple figures would enable the results achieved to be compared with the targets:

— the yearly total number of cases of neonatal tetanus occurring in the entire district compared with the target for that year
— the yearly number of cases of neonatal tetanus occurring in each village compared with the number that occurred in the previous year
— as calculated at the end of the plan period, the mean annual incidence of neonatal tetanus in each village (i.e. the total number of cases in each village during the 5-year plan period, divided by 5).

Comparing these figures on a year-to-year basis will show whether the district totals decrease in line with the targeted trend; whether any village has more cases of neonatal tetanus than previously and should therefore receive greater attention; and, at the end of the period, whether any village has always had a higher incidence of neonatal tetanus than others, which would suggest unequal accessibility, distribution or quality of services.

The time to make this comparison might be in the last quarter of each financial year, to allow for budgetary changes to be made for the following year. The task would fall on, say, the district nurse-midwife in charge of neonatal tetanus; the findings should be made available to the district management, preferably in the form of tables and written conclusions.

Judge the degree to which the results achieved have been of value

Once the measurements and comparisons have been made, the evaluation group must judge the value to the community of what has been achieved. In the example used here, this is a simple matter of whether the annual and total incidence of neonatal tetanus has been reduced to the targeted figure, and whether the distribution norm (e.g. no more than one case in each village) has been met. There may therefore be little more to discuss if the principle of 'management by exception' (see Part I, Chapter 1) is applied. However, it is usually advisable to hold a meeting of those who planned and produced the services and of members of the concerned communities to discuss the results and how they were obtained, even when an objective or target has been achieved. For instance, it might have been possible to achieve the target sooner with no additional effort, or to achieve better results with the same effort. The experience gained in achieving a target or objective is likely to be valuable for other programmes.

When results fall below what was expected, the reasons must be explored and analysed. The analysis should take place before the annual report is made, so that remedial action may be proposed to the higher or supervising level. Discussions should involve a member of the health team, a health volunteer from the villages or areas where the shortfalls occurred, and a representative of the community concerned.

Decide what to do next

On the principle of 'management by exception', no new decisions are needed when targets and objectives have been satisfactorily achieved, except to continue as before. Of course, the objectives and targets may have been set at too low a level, and this should be considered when they have proved easy to achieve. When achievement has not been satisfactory, however, one type of decision may be to investigate thoroughly the causes of the shortfall by means of assessment, appraisal of staff performance, management audit (see Section 3.5) or otherwise. A different kind of decision might be to reassign staff or resources to strengthen the effort where needed. These decisions are for the team leader to make; they should be made promptly and communicated to all concerned for immediate action.

3.2 Evaluating work progress

Work progress is evaluated in order to measure the efficiency of the health team, i.e. to find out whether the team completed the work that was assigned to it in order to reach its targets (quantity), whether the work was of the expected quality and was carried out on time, and whether the budget was overspent or not.

The basic questions to be asked are:

● Are the results those that were intended?
● If not, why not?

Evaluation for efficiency covers the same five steps as were discussed in Section 3.1:

— deciding what aspects of the programme to evaluate for efficiency, and how to measure or assess efficiency
— collecting the information needed to measure the achievements
— comparing the results with the norms and targets
— judging the value of the work achieved
— deciding what to do next.

Decide what to evaluate and select measures of operational efficiency

Normally, a plan of action outlines the work of the health team. It lists the necessary activities (services to be delivered, development work, and support tasks), indicates what they should achieve, who should perform them and when each should take place, and shows how each activity would relate to the others.

If this has been done, it will not be difficult to monitor and evaluate the team's efficiency. The questions to be asked are:

- Were the planned activities completed?
- Did they achieve their targets?
- Did they do so on time and with the assigned staff and other resources?

If the plan of action did not specify the team's activities, and much of the work has been completed, the team leader must decide whether there is a valid reason for attempting to evaluate the team's performance for efficiency. If there is such a reason, those responsible for evaluation should list all the activities that should have been carried out and what they should have achieved. This is a useful exercise only if it enables the evaluators to determine which resources were critical for the success of the activities or, if the activities did not achieve their targets, which critical resources were lacking. Since it will be possible to examine only a few activities among many, they must be carefully chosen. The criterion for choosing the activities would be, for example, that they must be completed before many later activities can begin, or that they must use a large amount of critical resources.

For instance:

> To control neonatal tetanus in Jaya District, the three critically important preceding activities are: TBAs to be retrained in sterile handling of the umbilical cord (a development activity); mothers to be immunized at antenatal clinics (a service activity); messages on prevention of neonatal tetanus to be spread to the people (a support activity). The first is selected because retraining is critical and trainers are a critical resource in short supply, and the second and third because mothers must be motivated before they demand immunization and choose to be delivered by retrained TBAs.

The activities to be evaluated should be selected from among those listed at least one year before a report is due. They should be selected by the staff member in charge of neonatal tetanus — probably the public health nurse-midwife. The selected activities should be reviewed with those who will later take part in collecting information about them and analysing it, to ensure that it will be possible to obtain the necessary information from the field.

Collect the necessary information

The results of activities (operational outputs) may be measured in many ways. Thus, in the above example, 'retrained TBAs' may be measured as the number trained per month, the total number available in each village, or the number who have passed some qualifying test. The operational output 'mothers immunized' may be expressed as a number or as a percentage of pregnant women in each village or in the district. The operational output 'message spread' may be measured at the source (newspapers, radio, etc.), at the receiving end (individual mothers reached) or at some intermediate point (village heads transmitting the information). Achievements should normally be measured in the same terms as those in which the targets were set, or at least in terms that can be related to the set targets. When there is a choice, the achievements to be measured should be those that can be more easily (or more cheaply) measured, provided that ease of measurement does not result in unreliable information.

For instance:

> In Jaya District, it was decided to use three variables for measuring the work progress of a health team: (a) the yearly number of immunized pregnant women, expressed as a percentage of the total number of pregnant women; (b) the yearly *additional* number of TBAs retrained, as a percentage of the total practising; and (c) the proportion of village heads transmitting five or more messages. This entails the continuous monitoring of immunizations at all antenatal clinics and estimating the total number of pregnancies in one year; recording newly retrained TBAs at each successive course; estimating the number of TBAs practising at some point in time; and surveying all the village heads once a year.

This example deals with the information to be collected. The three tasks of collecting, recording, and reporting and processing would be assigned to the staff in charge of services, training and support activities respectively. The timing would be, for example, monthly collection and reporting, quarterly processing and yearly summing-up.

Compare achievements with norms and targets

So that achievements may be compared with norms and targets, the available or collected information should be tabulated, to show the results of training, immunization and communication activities against the corresponding norms and targets. Assuming yearly evaluation, such tables should present results for the completed year. Moreover, to keep track of where activities took place, results should be presented for each village or area.

If the norms and targets have been expressed as rates or ratios, the tables must show the denominators as well as the numerators. In the above example the denominators are the numbers of pregnant women in the villages and the numbers of registered or practising TBAs, and the numerators are the numbers of women immunized and the numbers of TBAs retrained. Then it will be possible to express the rate of immunization coverage and the proportion of TBAs retrained.

To monitor the progress of activities that must be carried out before certain specified dates, it may be necessary to prepare tables each month to show the position at the end of each month or quarter.

For instance:

> For Jaya District, such tables might show whether the TBA retraining programme had achieved its target in the district as a whole, in which villages the training of practising TBAs had been completed, in which it was still continuing, and where it had yet to start. Similarly, for immunization, successive tables should show the district coverage, the coverage of each village, where the targets had been reached, where they had not been reached, and where activities had yet to begin. The communication of messages to the public should also be presented in a table showing which villages had been well covered, which poorly covered and which not yet covered.

On the basis of such tables, the results can also be recorded on maps to show the geographical pattern of work progress and of target achievement. This can help reveal factors that assist or hinder the team's performance.

Judge the degree to which norms have been met

If information has been analysed and presented in tables as described above, each target can be reviewed both separately and in relation to the others. The recording of results on maps helps the evaluators to determine how far norms and targets have been met in the district as a whole. Successive monthly or quarterly tables can show to what extent targets are being achieved within the time specified for them.

It may be found that one of the activities being measured appears satisfactory in relation to the corresponding target, but that the other activities have lagged behind.

For instance:

> In some villages of Jaya District, it is found that the training of TBAs and the spread of messages by village heads are up to expectation (targeted level), but that the immunization coverage is far below the district average.

Here it may be useful to study the relation between these three activities in other villages. Such a study may show that a group of villages, all close to each other, have the same kind of results.

For instance:

> A number of villages in north-east Jaya present the same picture: good message-spread, satisfactory immunization coverage, but no training activities.

This suggests that something is interfering with or taking the place of retraining of TBAs. The situation should be investigated in discussion with the health workers concerned and with the people of the villages. It should then be possible to judge the results on the basis of a clear understanding of the local situation.

In judging work progress and operational output it is also helpful to take into account the results of the programme (i.e. its effectiveness), as discussed in Section 3.1 above. Operational outputs are not ends in themselves but rather means towards successful results, e.g. no cases of neonatal tetanus. Analysis and discussion should show whether good results are necessarily the outcome of good achievement and, conversely, whether good work progress automatically means good results. It might also show whether one activity (say, immunization) is more frequently associated with good results than others.

This kind of analysis is extremely important: adequate staff and time should be assigned to it. When the information provided in the tables is reliable and valid, the time spent on interpreting and understanding it is well spent. Participants in the analysis will learn from it (See Part II, Chapter 3, Section 3.6, "Training staff"), and the whole health team should study it. Conclusions should be communicated to the decision-makers who control the programme at higher level, and to participating staff and village heads or health committees, in preparation for the next and final step.

Decide what to do next

Two types of decision are required at this stage — whether performance must be further assessed, and whether the programme needs to be improved.

For further in-depth assessment of performance, the team leader may assign one staff member to study the available material as a means of appraising staff performance (see Section 3.3 below). As regards improving the programme, the team leader may await the results of appraisal of staff performance, or may judge it right to introduce certain changes in the programme.

For instance:

> In Jaya District, the team leader may:
>
> — schedule work in such a way that the three component activities (training, information and immunization) are coordinated, i.e. ensure that, in villages where one component has been achieved (e.g. TBA training), the others are also carried out and vice versa.
> — change some of the TBA's work instructions, and redesign the corresponding retraining curriculum, so that immunization of pregnant women receives the necessary attention, or offer some incentives to the TBAs to increase the demand for immunization.

3.3 Appraising staff performance

It will be recalled that the main purpose of evaluation is to learn from experience and thus to improve the programme. Staff performance is appraised in order that staff may learn from experience and therefore improve or maintain satisfactory levels of performance.

One specific purpose of appraisal of staff performance should be to enable decisions to be made about the learning needs of staff. The two basic questions to be asked are very similar to those involved in evaluating achievements and work progress, but are concerned here with staff performance:

- Are the results as good as they could be?
- If not, why not?

The appraisal process also involves the following five steps:

— deciding what aspects of performance to appraise
— collecting the information needed to measure performance
— comparing the results with relevant norms
— judging the degree to which norms are met
— deciding what to do next.

It should be emphasized, both to the appraiser and to the staff member whose performance is to be appraised, that performance appraisal is not intended to find fault with staff, even when results fall short of what was intended. Rather, appraisal should be understood and appreciated as *the* way to help each staff member perform efficiently and to feel gratified when he or she achieves the intended results.

As with other evaluation activities, there must be rules that state who is responsible for making the appraisal, the date when the appraisal is due, the period covered by the appraisal, the information needed to make the appraisal, and the information needed from the appraisal (e.g. a performance *appraisal report*).

Decide what to appraise and select indicators of performance

Three documents should normally specify all the functions, tasks or activities that should be the subject of performance appraisal. These are:

— the job description
— a work plan (or work assignment, work schedule, or work instructions)
— technical procedure manuals.

The job description, discussed in Part II, Chapter 3:

— lists the functions that a staff member is expected to perform (e.g. providing services, conducting research, undertaking surveys, training students, maintaining equipment, keeping accounts)
— states to whom (the supervisor) the staff member is accountable for the performance of these functions
— states for whom (subordinates) the staff member is responsible in the performance of their functions

— indicates with whom (peers, partners) the staff member is to coordinate in the performance of joint functions.

The work plan (described in Part III, Chapter 4):

— assigns the staff member's activities and tasks
— describes in detail the services a staff member has to deliver
— specifies the extent of the services to be provided (and often the people who should receive them)
— states where these services have to be delivered
— states when the services are to be delivered.

Technical procedure manuals usually describe in some detail how particular tasks with a high technical content are to be performed; examples of such tasks include immunizing, conducting workshops, writing health educational materials.

When job descriptions, work plans and technical procedure manuals have been properly prepared, are up to date and are followed correctly, performance appraisal is straightforward. When they have not been prepared in detail, however, performance appraisal begins with ascertaining the description of staff functions, activities and tasks from management, staff, subordinates or users of the services, as appropriate.

It will be rare to find complete understanding and agreement between those directly concerned, and this makes performance appraisal difficult and its conclusions indefinite.

In either case, the appraiser should select a limited number of tasks and activities (up to five, say) as a basis for the appraisal of staff performance. These should be tasks and activities that make the greatest contribution to the health team's efficiency and effectiveness, such as organizing, coordinating, monitoring and controlling.

For instance:

>In the case of the nurse-midwife in charge of controlling neonatal tetanus in Jaya District, the functions, activities and tasks she performs in that programme are:
>
>organization
>— coordination
>— monitoring
>— control.

Her performance should be appraised against:

(a) the results achieved
(b) the services delivered
(c) the TBAs retrained
(d) the messages reaching the community.

Thus, her performance would be appraised as follows:

For organization against (c) and (d), the timely completion of planned courses for TBAs and the diffusion of messages.

For coordination against (b), (c) and (d), the proportion of villages reaching the targets for services, retraining of TBAs, and diffusion of messages.

For monitoring against (a) and (b), the availability of up-to-date statistics on incidence of neonatal tetanus and on immunizations, from all parts of the district.

For control against management of resources and supplies, so that work is not impeded by shortages of funds or vaccine, for instance.

As is clear from this example, it is assumed that the management functions of the nurse-midwife are critical to programme success. In other situations and programmes, the technical or public-relations functions might be more suitable for performance appraisal.

On appointment of a staff member, and annually as part of the planning process, the team leader and other team members should together agree on norms and targets so that there is no doubt about the performance expected of both the team as a whole and its individual members.

Collect the necessary information

The information required to measure performance may be available from routine records or may need to be collected. Thus, in the above example, the necessary information would include dates of completion of planned courses and of diffusion of messages, the proportion of pregnant women immunized and the number of cases of neonatal tetanus occurring in the period under review, and the number of villages where targets for services, training and the diffusion of messages had and had not been reached.

For instance:

> There would be routine records of dates of completion of TBA retraining courses, of villages reaching the target levels for services, and of how far the statistics lag behind, but a special enquiry might be needed to obtain details of diffusion of messages by village heads, on work stoppages, and on shortages of funds or vaccine, which may not be automatically recorded.

This kind of special task is best performed by the staff themselves, as part of the regular monitoring of service and other activities for which they are primarily responsible. In delegating this task to them, management enables staff to be the first to learn of their own successes and failures, and to adjust their performance when necessary.

Compare observations with norms and standards

In most instances, performance is appraised in relation to operational or time targets, and appraisal relies primarily on the routine monitoring of programme activities; comparison of intended and actual performance does not therefore cause special difficulties.

For instance:

> Excerpt from the 1992 performance appraisal for the public health nurse in Jaya District:
>
> *"Organizational performance*: All four courses for TBAs in her health area were completed as scheduled and with the target number of trainees.
>
> *Coordination performance*: In 1992, three villages reached target levels of the three activities that she coordinates, against an expected six.
>
> *Monitoring performance*: Operational statistics are up to date, but statistics on births and deaths are one month behind.
>
> *Control performance*: No work stoppages occurred during the year in her health area."

It is usually argued that, to avoid bias, this task should be performed by management and not by the staff member. However, when the management functions are shared by all staff, and when norms of performance and targets have been agreed upon by the staff concerned and the team leader, a staff member's performance appraisal may be entrusted to the staff member (subject to review and approval by the responsible officer). The timing should satisfy the regulations of the national administration.

Judge the degree to which staff performance meets required standards

The comparison of performance with norms and targets needs interpretation for two reasons. First, not all aspects of staff performance are equally important and, second, success in one area must be balanced against failure in another. The evaluator needs to exercise careful judgement here and may need additional information and results of tests of knowledge and skill before reaching a conclusion.

For instance:

> *Subject*: Performance of the public health nurse
>
> *Conclusions of team leader*: The public health nurse has proved to be a good organizer; she has kept herself informed of work progress, thus exercising firm control over the programme. She would benefit from support in coordination tasks, based on her own assessment (on attached questionnaire) of her:
>
> — oral communication ability
> — problem-solving ability
> — ability to conduct meetings
> — ability to resolve conflict.

To make this judgement, the team leader must have considered some of the possible causes of the apparently poor coordination performance of the staff member, obtained some informal explanation for this shortcoming, and concluded that her coordinating ability could be improved by training. However, the team leader wants the staff member to identify her priority needs.

It is evident from this example that judgement is a team leader's responsibility. However, such judgement should be made in open discussion with the staff.

Decide what to do next

As seen above, one possible decision following an appraisal of staff performance concerns further training. This might require further analysis of events or of the range of ability of the staff member. Such a decision, however, would often affect programme activities as well, for instance in re-assigning certain tasks to other staff with the requisite skills or abilities, strengthening some coordination or control mechanism, or simply communicating certain information to the concerned people. The important thing that any decision must show is that appraisal of staff performance is not intended to work *against* staff but rather to *promote* the team's efficiency, effectiveness and, ultimately, job satisfaction.

The responsibility for such decisions rests with the team leader, but the wise team leader will always make sure that the staff concerned take part in reaching the decisions.

3.4 Evaluating use of resources

Elsewhere in this guide the concept and methods of monitoring and control have been introduced as management tools for reaching day-to-day decisions about the allocation of resources. What, then, is the purpose of evaluating, as opposed to monitoring and controlling, the use of resources? In this context, evaluation differs from monitoring in being concerned with *how* the resources used relate to results achieved over a period of, say, one year, with the aim of answering the following questions:

● Could some resources achieve better results or outputs?
● Could some results be achieved with fewer resources?

The questions are actually two sides of the same coin: in management terms, the first deals with 'cost-effectiveness' and the second with 'cost-efficiency'.

Some practical aspects of these concepts are considered in this section, following the same five steps as were used in the preceding sections:

— deciding what aspects of resource use to evaluate
— collecting the necessary information
— comparing resource use with norms and standards
— judging the degree to which norms have been met
— deciding what to do next.

Decide what aspects of resource use to evaluate

One of the most useful measures of resource use is the 'amount of a specified resource used to deliver some unit of work or achieve some unit of result'. This is less complicated than it sounds, and could be equated with saying "My motorcycle runs for 100 kilometres on 2 litres of petrol", which is an example of 'unit cost' in terms of petrol consumption.

To select 'unit costs' for evaluating the use of resources in relation to results and outputs, it is necessary to identify critical results or outputs and the resources consumed in achieving or producing them. This, again, is the application of the principle of 'management by exception': looking for the most important of the things that need doing and doing it first.

For instance:

> In Jaya District, control of neonatal tetanus is measured by the number of cases prevented; the most immediately relevant operational output is immunization of pregnant women; money is the scarcest of the resources available to the health team. Thus, the cost of preventing one case of neonatal tetanus and the cost of one immunization would be suitable measures of cost-efficiency.

In principle, the plan should specify that the programme would be monitored and evaluated for cost-efficiency on this basis.

Collect the necessary information

Previous chapters have discussed the monitoring and reporting of results and operational outputs, and management of funds has been described in Part III. Certain difficulties may be encountered in putting these methods into practice, however. For instance, with reference to the example that has now been used many times, TBAs may be trained in some places but not in others; in some places fewer than five messages may be diffused and in others more; immunization coverage may be low in some places and high in others. For these reasons, the cost — and effectiveness — of the programme will vary from village to village, and it will therefore be of no value to estimate unit costs for the district as a whole. Measurement of resources used (expressed here in terms of cost) should take full account of these variations; it is to be hoped that the extra effort this will entail will yield extra information.

For instance:

> In Jaya District, unit costs of immunization should be measured:
>
> — by incorporating the costs of TBA training and the costs of message diffusion, where these activities occur
> — by excluding these costs where they do not.

Collecting information about costs in this way will allow more valid comparisons to be made. Cost measurement, however, is an accountancy task, for which few, if any, health staff will be trained. Where it is intended from the outset to evaluate resource use, accountancy skills should be brought into the team on a more or less continuous basis throughout the implementation of the programme.

Compare resource use with norms and standards

Norms and standards for the use of resources cannot be laid down in advance; they will emerge as a result of the evaluation. In answering the question "Can more be done with these resources?", the highest observed output per unit of resource will become the norm; conversely, the question "Could we do as well with fewer resources?" will yield a norm equal to the lowest cost per unit of output.

For instance:

> In Jaya District, the unit cost of immunization in villages where TBAs are trained and messages are diffused is $2.50, and coverage is 75%. Where only immunization is provided, the unit cost varies from $2.10 to $2.30 according to the coverage achieved, but coverage never exceeds 60%.

Costs and coverages are compared, and careful judgement must be used by the evaluator. The task requires time, and skills and information that are not easily acquired; evaluation of this kind would normally require support from the health administration.

Judge the degree to which norms have been met

When the cheapest approach to achieving a particular result has been determined, a basis is created for examining other approaches. Similarly, when the highest output possible within stated resource limits has been determined, it is possible to discuss how lower outputs were achieved. Considerations of this sort are essential for improving programme strategy, but who undertakes them, where and when, will depend on an individual country's administrative structure.

Decide on future use of resources

Of the decisions that are likely to result from such considerations, one might be to drop a particular component of the programme if it proved to be adding a lot to costs in relation to what it achieved. A second type of decision might be to set less ambitious coverage targets for the future if no extra resources could be provided. Yet a third type of decision would be to try to persuade authorities to increase the budget to enable the health team to meet its targets.

Decisions of this kind are usually made at levels higher than that of the health team, but health teams should be aware of the usefulness of the evaluation to the decision-making process and should be encouraged to ask relevant questions.

3.5 The management audit

A management audit is a method of reviewing management activities; it is a checklist of questions relating to management. Management audit can be used as a tool by health workers with management functions to examine their own successes and failures, or it can be used by supervisors to assess the management efficiency of an organization. The process can be highly complex, covering every aspect of management organization, or very simple, asking only a few carefully constructed questions to reveal the general standard of organization and efficiency.

A management audit is a summary of all operational control processes. When the management audit is repeated, the results of action taken after the previous audit are noted.

An example of a simple management audit for a rural health unit can be found below. This covers some of the management functions described in Parts I, II, III and IV.

Example: Management audit for a rural health unit

Under the date of audit, write Y (yes) or N (no) opposite each statement.

1) Planning and organization	Date	Action	Date	Action
The health centre has one or more defined objectives	2.1.93 Y	Immunize 400 children	3.1.94 Y	Completed
These objectives are known to the health team				
Regular staff meetings are held				
A year-plan has been written and displayed				
There is a weekly timetable				
Staff duties are listed on a roster				
District activities are scheduled in advance				
Changes in rosters, schedules or other events are clearly communicated to the health team				

2) Personnel

Each member of the team has a written job description
Each staff member knows to whom to report and from whom to receive instructions
The team leader delegates work whenever possible
On-the-job training is aided in different ways — by supervision, discussion, books or demonstrations
The team leader acknowledges good work
The work provides opportunities for initiative and responsibility
Supervision takes the form of educating and helping rather than criticizing
Workers are using the skills for which they were trained
Team members show concern for the welfare of patients

3) Resources

The account ledgers are in order and up to date
The petty-cash balance sheet is correct
There is sufficient equipment
The stock ledger is balanced and corresponds to the store shelves and inventories
Drug issues are recorded and reviewed
The 'A/B' shelf system is used for vital drugs
There are minimum queues and 'bottlenecks' in the outpatient clinic
There are adequate and clearly marked maps of the district
The transport system is well maintained

	Date	Action	Date	Action
4) District and public				
There is a health-centre committee of people within the area				
Efforts are made to educate the public in health				
The health needs of the public are identified and discussed				
Health goals and activities relate to public health needs				
The following health activities are expanding:				
— maternal and child clinics				
— immunization				
— nutrition programme				
— sanitation programme				
5) Control system				
There are monthly statistical reports				
There is an annual report				
The patient registers are clear and up to date				
Patient records can be found when necessary				
Copies of letters are made and filed				
There is an index of files and registers				
There is a well-kept log in the transport vehicle				
There is a method for discovering discrepancies in drug usage				

Exercises

Exercise 60 (IV.1) Household health survey

Objective: To be able to collect, analyse and use baseline information for planning primary health care.

Individual work

List the information needed for planning a primary health care service, and adapt a household health survey form from the example shown on pages 275–278, to suit your requirements.

Group work

Review the information requirements specified by the health workers, and the household survey forms they designed, and finalize a single form that satisfies the more important requirements. Decide on the survey population and method, and assign areas to each health worker.

Individual work

Survey the households assigned to you, interview heads of households, and record the information collected.

Group work

Compile *demographic* information, such as:

— total population in surveyed area
— distribution by age and sex
— distribution by household size
— birth rates (live, still)
— death rates (by age and sex if sufficient numbers)

Compile *health* information, such as:

— mean height, weight, arm circumference of children at age 5 years
— mean number of episodes of illness recalled over past year, and frequency of main symptoms (as percentages of all episodes)
— mean number of disabilities at time of survey, and frequency by type and duration

— important health problems, as stated by heads of households
— care practices (percentage of people using formal health services, other health services, no outside help)
— health-care expenditure (on services, drugs, transport).

Classify the demographic and health information according to head-of-household status, recorded environmental factors, etc.

Exercise 61 (IV.1) Priority health problems of communities

Objective: To be able to recognize and select priority health problems of the community for planning primary health care services.

Individual work

Review the list of selection criteria shown on pages 284–285 and adapt it to local needs if necessary. List community health problems, including those stated by heads of households in the household survey (Exercise 60). Then check each important health problem against the criteria, and assign a priority ranking according to how many criteria each problem satisfies (the more criteria satisfied, the higher the priority).

Group work

Review the proposed selection criteria, discuss their implications and agree on a common list. Then check the priority problems, as listed by the health workers or stated by the surveyed heads of households, against the agreed criteria.

Assign a common priority ranking of community health problems. Compare the priority list with official health policy statements, note points of agreement, and discuss and decide what should be done about points of divergence.

Exercise 62 (IV.1) Selecting a strategy

Objective: To be able to analyse possible obstacles to the achievement of objectives, and to select a feasible strategy for implementation.

Many targets may be set, but they are not all equally likely to be reached. The health team must analyse possible obstacles so as to retain the strategy most likely to succeed.

This exercise is about alternative maternal and child health (MCH) actions, and the related operational targets, designed to reduce infant and maternal mortality over a period of 5 years in a community of 5000 inhabitants with a birth rate of 40/1000.

Individual work

Study the actions and service targets listed below, which have been prepared for achieving the objective.

Action	Targets	No. of services/year
(a) One antenatal visit to the health centre by	100% of pregnant women	= 2000 visits
(b) Three antenatal visits in villages to	50% of pregnant women	= 3000 visits
(c) Supervised home delivery of	80% of pregnant women	= 1600 deliveries
(d) Contraception practised in	25% of households	= 1000 visits
(e) Nutritional education sessions in villages for	60% of pregnant women	= 120 sessions

What are the obstacles to each action? List the obstacles in order of importance. When you have studied all the actions, judge which of the 10 possible combinations of two actions is most feasible. Indicate what steps will be necessary to carry out the two actions you select.

Group work

Review and tabulate the lists of obstacles to each action, and the estimated importance of each. Agree on a common list in order of relative importance for each action.

From the list, compare the feasibility of the possible sets of two actions, and retain the most feasible.

Exercise 63 (IV.1) Scheduling primary health care activities

Objective: To be able to plan the activities necessary to reach strategy targets and to overcome the anticipated obstacles.

Individual work

An MCH strategy selected for one community (as in Exercise 62) consists of:

— one antenatal visit to the health centre before the fifth month of pregnancy for 100% of pregnant women in the villages = 2000 visits a year
— home delivery supervised by 100 trained TBAs in 80% of cases = 16 deliveries a year by each TBA
— monthly nutrition education sessions in all villages, for 60% of the women = 120 sessions a year

Review the list of possible obstacles to the implementation of this strategy (from Exercise 62), and write down all the *activities* the health team will have to undertake to achieve the targets *and* overcome the obstacles. Number the activities.

Take one or several activities; assign a responsible staff member to each activity, state how *frequently* the staff member must perform the activity in a month, and *how much time* (in hours) the staff member will have to spend on the activity.

Think how you should present this information to show the sequence and interdependence of staff activities.

Group work

Review the lists of activities suggested by health workers and agree on a common list.

Decide which activities are required once only (e.g. development activities) and which need to be repeated (e.g. service activities), and agree on the frequency of each activity.

Discuss and agree on assignments among the various members of the team, then review the estimates of staff time required for each activity.

Discuss how to present the information on activities and finalize a schedule containing the essentials of the information.

Exercise 64 (IV.1) Estimating costs

Objective: To be able to estimate the various costs of a strategy so as to assess the adequacy of the resources available to implement it.

Cost is the amount of a given resource consumed.[1] This exercise focuses on a component (c) of the strategy outlined in Exercise 62, namely *supervised home delivery of 1600 women in 10 villages.*

Individual work

List the five principal resources used in health work, and show in a table which resources are required for each activity related to home delivery attended by a midwife or TBA (see Exercise 63).

Focus on one resource, namely the staff time required. Assume that one health centre midwife and 100 TBAs are the only staff involved, and that the frequency of each activity, and the estimates of staff time required for each activity, are as shown in the solution to Exercise 63. Calculate the total midwife and TBA time required.

Is there sufficient staff time available to implement the strategy?

Group work

Review the proposed lists of resources consumed in health work, and agree on a short list of five. Review which resources are used in each activity, and discuss the significance of staff time as a resource.

Review how the health workers calculated the total staff time required to implement supervised home delivery. Select by discussion the 'best' method and record it for further reference.

Compare the results obtained by the health workers and find a common answer by using the 'best' method.

Discuss the feasibility of supervised home delivery on the basis of staff time used compared with staff time available.

---

[1] Money is only one resource (see page 300).

Discuss what could, and ought to, be done when it is concluded that some strategy component is not feasible within the available staff time.

Note: Repeat this exercise for other types of resources, until feasibility can be assessed with regard to funds.

Exercise 65 (IV.2) Coordinating

Objective: To be able to name, design and use simple ways to coordinate health work.

Individual work

Activities have been scheduled for the achievement of strategy targets (Exercise 63). Now study the following example of a monthly MCH activity schedule.

Activity schedule	Staff	Frequency (per month)	Time/unit activity	Resources
Service				
(1) Antenatal home visit	Midwife	125–175	15 min	MCH kit
(2) Supervised home delivery	TBA	15	8 hours	Sterile delivery kit
(3) Nutrition education for pregnant women	Midwife	10 sessions	2 hours	Transport Charts Demonstration equipment
Development				
(4) Write educational material	Midwife	1 session	2 hours	Nutrition literature
(5) Train TBAs	Midwife TBAs	1 session	2 hours	Learning materials Transport
Support				
(6) Maintain TBA kits	Midwife TBAs	1	15 min	Expendable supplies
Information				
(7) Update family records	Midwife	30	15 min	Family health cards
Management				
(8) Supervision visit	Midwife TBA	10	30 min	Checklist

Total time per month   Midwife: 73 hours
                         TBA: 127 hours

As coordinator of these activities, indicate:

— which activities take place only in the villages, which only at the
  health centre and which in both places;
— which activities can be performed together during one visit to a village;
— other activities that need to be coordinated.

If you could add *one* activity to this schedule to make it more complete and
responsive to health needs, what would it be?

Group work

Review the statements of the health workers, discuss any differences
between them, and agree on a common solution to the exercise.

Review the list of coordination mechanisms for generating and communicating decisions and for achieving agreement of the *who, what, how, when*
and *where* of coordination.

Review the list of coordination instruments — written documents — that
help to achieve coordination, clarify who is responsible for issuing them
and to whom each should be addressed. (Check where each of these
documents is referred to in this book.)

Exercise 66 (IV.2) Monitoring work progress

Objective: To be able to say what needs to be monitored in the work, and to
design and use simple methods of monitoring work progress.

To *monitor* is, simply, to watch for what is on or behind schedule and what
is or is not progressing as expected.

Individual work

In the situation described and analysed in Exercise 65, you wish to keep
yourself informed about how well work proceeds against the schedule.

What needs monitoring? Suggest a few aspects of the work you believe
should be watched carefully (say, one aspect per activity). For each item of

information state *who* should:

— obtain it
— compile and analyse it
— record findings
— report findings (and to whom).

Then explain *how* monitoring takes place in respect of two items chosen from the above list.

Group work

Review what health workers have chosen for monitoring, activity by activity, and agree on a common checklist of what needs to be monitored.

Where necessary, discuss the reasons *why* these aspects of the work should be monitored. Record the agreed reasons.

Review the assignment of responsibility for monitoring, step by step — collection, recording, compilation, and reporting. Discuss the current assignments at the health centre, and make suggestions for improvement.

Finally, review how the monitoring process should take place at the health centre, critically discussing the current situation with a view to suggesting improvements.

Note: This exercise may be repeated for one or more aspects of primary health care work.

Exercise 67 (IV.2) Monitoring performance

Objective: To be able to say what activities and tasks need monitoring in staff performance and to assign simple ways of monitoring.

Individual work

Review your job description and the service work you are doing. For each service activity and task you perform, certain norms of performance may have been set; write down those you are aware of (e.g. technical norms, behaviour norms, management norms).

Then check which activities and tasks are routinely monitored, either by yourself or by someone else. Are these the same activities and tasks for which norms or standards of performance have been set? Prepare yourself to discuss this topic.

Group work

Review the health workers' activities and tasks for which there are norms/standards of performance and record them. (Whenever possible, refer to a written document.) Then check all activities and tasks that are routinely monitored, and record who does the monitoring.

Discuss how performance is monitored at present — for example, are valid norms of performance used and are staff members clear about the purpose of monitoring performance. Determine activities and tasks for which norms, or new norms, should be set, and which should be routinely monitored. Record the conclusions reached and submit them to the supervisor for consideration.

Exercise 68 (IV.2) Monitoring achievement

Objective: To be able to state the targets that have been set for the team and to monitor individual programmes directed towards meeting them.

The monitoring of work progress and performance helps ensure that targets are met. The monitoring of achievement shows the extent to which targets are being met.

Individual work

Refer to the activity schedule proposed in Exercise 63.

List the specific information you would need in order to monitor achievement in all relevant activities in the situation described. Check that each item of information can be matched with the stated targets.

Name the staff member responsible for collecting each item of information. Suggest the frequency with which each item should be collected (daily, weekly, monthly, etc.).

State to which staff member each collected item of information should be sent in the described situation.

Then list the targets towards which your own work is directed, and repeat the above steps in respect of the different activities. Review your current practice in monitoring your own achievement against what should be done, and prepare yourself to discuss this topic.

Group work

Invite one individual to describe the monitoring of achievement in the MCH situation under consideration.

Review the health workers' descriptions of the process of monitoring achievement in their different work areas.

Discuss the gap — if any — between current practice and desired procedure. Consolidate a list of the additional information that should be collected, who should collect it, and to whom it should be directed, so as to perform a useful monitoring of achievement.

Exercise 69 (IV.2) Controlling deficiencies

Objective: To be able to name the control decisions that follow monitoring, to explain how they are made, and to execute them.

Observing work progress and how the health team functions, and monitoring how health workers perform, do not automatically improve effectiveness or efficiency. This requires knowing what needs to be improved and deciding to do it — in other words, controlling deficiencies.

Individual work

Consider the following findings obtained from monitoring the work described in Exercise 65:

Activity 1	75 pregnant women attended the antenatal clinic last month
Activity 2	20 TBAs attended fewer than 10 deliveries each last year. 30 TBAs attended more than 15 deliveries each last year. 50 TBAs attended between 10 and 15 deliveries each. No complications were reported by any TBA.
Activity 3	In four villages very few women attend nutrition education sessions.

Activity 4	Preparation of educational materials is one month behind schedule.
Activity 5	10% of TBAs have not attended any learning session.
Activity 6	Information on the cost of supplies is not available at the health centre.
Activity 7	Deliveries are not usually recorded in family health records until the subsequent pregnancy. Birth weights of babies are unknown.
Activity 8	A midwife has made supervision visits to TBAs in nine villages in each of the past three months.

Note the deficiencies in the work monitored, and list what you would do to rectify them. Review your list of proposed remedial actions to decide *who* would take the necessary action. Are those who monitor work progress, staff performance, and achievement also responsible for taking remedial action?

Group work

Review the health workers' lists of deficiencies, discuss differences in interpretation, and agree on a common list.

Discuss and record who monitors the work and decides what the deficiencies are.

Review the suggestions for remedying the deficiencies and agree on the best possible action.

Assign responsibility for deciding on and implementing remedial action, and compare the lists of those who are responsible for monitoring and those who should take the remedial action. In each case, discuss whether any outside decision is required and, if so, from whom.

Conclude by recording all the control decisions and subsequent remedial actions that can be taken by the staff concerned without the need for outside intervention.

Exercise 70 (IV.3) Supervision

Objective: To be able to state what to expect from supervision during a field visit and to prepare for such a visit.

Supervision should help those who are supervised to perform better. Staff should be ready to acknowledge their need for help, just as the supervisor should recognize that giving help is a part of the supervision function.

Individual work

Read the checklist given below and decide which statements truly apply to the existing situation in the health facility.

For those statements that are not true of your situation, ask yourself whether or not you feel concerned. If you do feel concern about particular deficiencies, try to decide what could be done to remedy the problem. Record in a few words what you would expect from a supervisor's visit to enable you to cope better with specific problems.

Group your needs in a few suitable categories and prepare yourself for a discussion on this topic.

Group work

Review each statement in the checklist to discover the health workers' perception of the functioning of their health facilities and the extent to which they agree with one another. Record the results.

Record those areas in which health workers express concern about deficiencies and the extent to which all or most of them share common concerns.

Then review and discuss individual needs for help, and as far as possible agree upon the most important. As needs for help are repeated, group them in a few categories as suggested by the health workers.

Prepare a detailed statement of needs as perceived by staff for submission to supervisors as a basis for discussing future supervision programmes in a staff meeting.

Checklist for supervision of managerial activities

1) *Planning and organization*

   The health centre has one or more identified objectives.
   These objectives are known to the health team.
   Regular staff meetings are held.

A year-plan has been written and displayed.
There is a weekly timetable.
Staff duties are listed on a roster.
District activities are scheduled in advance.
Changes in rosters, schedules or other events are clearly communicated to the health team.

2) *Personnel*

Each member of the team has a written job description.
Each staff member knows to whom to report and from whom to receive instructions.
The team leader delegates work wherever possible.
On-the-job training is aided in different ways — by discussion, books or demonstrations.
Good work is acknowledged by the team leader.
Opportunity exists for initiative and responsibility in the work.
Supervision takes the form of educating and helping, not criticizing.
Workers are using the skills for which they were trained.
Team members show concern for the welfare of patients.

3) *Resources*

The account ledgers are in order and up to date.
The petty-cash balance sheet is correct.
There is sufficient equipment.
The stock ledger is balanced and corresponds to the store shelves and inventories.
Drug issues are recorded and reviewed.
The A/B shelf system is used for vital drugs.
There are minimum queues and 'bottlenecks' in the outpatient clinic.
There are adequate and clearly marked maps of the district.
The transport system is well maintained.

4) *District and public*

There is a health centre committee made up of people living in the area.
Efforts are made to educate the public in health.
The health needs of the public are identified and discussed.
The health goals and activities relate to public health needs.
The following health activities are expanding:

— maternal and child health clinics
— immunization
— nutrition programme
— sanitation programme.

5) *Control system*

There are monthly statistical reports.
There is an annual report.
The patient registers are clear and up to date.
Patient records can be found when necessary.
Carbon copies of letters are made and filed.
There is an index of files and registers.
There is a well-kept log in the transport vehicle.
There is a method to identify discrepancies in drug usage.

Exercise 71 (IV.3) Supervision and problem-solving

Objective: To be able, as a supervisor, to manage specific problems of implementation.

Individual work

The chairman of the village health committee complains to you about the village pharmacy. It seems that several village women who had gone to the pharmacy were told that the drugs they needed were not available, but that men had been supplied with the medicines they wanted. You take the opportunity of a supervisory visit to the area to try to solve the problem. Note that the health worker who maintains the village pharmacy was appointed by the village health committee and is therefore answerable to the committee and not to the health centre.

What would you do as a supervisor in such a situation? List the ideas as they occur to you, then list them in proper sequence, i.e. what you would do in preparation for the visit, during the visit, and after the visit.

For each activity you list, state *who* is involved, and who is *responsible* (e.g. chairman of the health committee, the committee, the midwife) and note one or more results or findings (e.g. stock ledger found to be up to date/poorly maintained/missing).

Depending on the results or findings, the situation may call for various follow-up activities. From your findings what follow-up activities would you suggest?

Group work

Discuss the nature of the reported situation, and agree on possible interpretations and causes.

Review the health workers' list of preparatory activities, their indications of who is responsible for each activity, and the expected results. Agree on a complete list of preparatory activities.

Then review the activities proposed during the supervisory visit; arrange them in such a way that they lead to a common understanding of the causes of the problem among the interested parties. Note who is responsible for each activity, and give examples of the products, findings or results of the activities.

Then review the suggested lists of follow-up activities and link each activity to specific findings. Discuss and agree on the expected results of, and the people responsible for, each follow-up activity.

Record the solutions of the exercise, and discuss the role of each health worker in problem-solving through supervision.

Exercise 72 (IV.3) Evaluation

Objective: To be able to analyse variations in incidence of an infectious disease throughout a district over a five-year period and to make interim evaluations of a control programme.

Individual or group work

Table I, below, shows the observed occurrence of neonatal tetanus in Jaya District, by village (A–AA) and year (1990–1994). In the base-year, 1990,

Table I. Cases of neonatal tetanus in villages of Jaya District, 1990–1994

Year	A	B	C	D	E	F	G	H	I	J	K	L	M	N	O	P	Q	R	S	T	U	V	W	X	Y	Z	AA	Total
1990	3	1	1	1	1	1	1	1	1	1	1																	13
1991	1		1	1	1		1		1	1	1				1	1					1							11
1992	1	1					1				1		1	1		1			1						1	1		10
1993				1							1	1		1		1		1			1				1	1		9
1994		1					1				1	1		1	1					1		1						8

13 cases were recorded (all in villages A to K) out of a total of 6500 births for the entire district — an incidence *rate* of 2 per 100 births.

Targets were set in 1990 for reducing the incidence rate of neonatal tetanus from 2 per 1000 births to 1 per 1000 in 1994. The expected number of births for 1995 is 7000. The target number of cases for that year is therefore 7 or less.

Comment on the fact that Table I shows no cases for villages L to AA in 1990. Why might this be?

Calculate the yearly total number of cases for the years 1991–1994. Is the observed trend what you expect?

Given the observed trend up to 1994, do you think that the target for 1995 will be met?

Study the yearly incidence of neonatal tetanus in villages A to K from 1990 to 1994. For each village calculate the mean yearly incidence (total number of recorded cases divided by 5) and name the three villages with the highest mean yearly incidence.

Comment on possible reasons for these three villages having a higher incidence.

What additional information would you need in order to decide whether the observed numbers represent a fall or a rise in incidence?

Table II shows the number of births registered in 1992 for each village. Calculate the mean yearly incidence *rate* of neonatal tetanus in villages A to K, dividing the mean number of cases by the number of registered births, and expressing the result per 1000 births. For instance in village J:

mean yearly incidence: 1
registered births (1994):   330
incidence rate 1 : 330   = 3 per 1000 births.

Table II. Births in villages of Jaya District, 1992

Village	A	B	C	D	E	Γ	G	H	I	J	K	L	M
Births	250	310	290	200	370	300	250	190	380	330	310	220	290

N	O	P	Q	R	S	T	U	V	W	X	Y	Z	AA
200	310	190	320	270	360	330	230	210	260	190	100	200	190

Pick out the three villages with the highest incidence rate. Are these the same as, or different from, the villages with the highest mean yearly incidence? Comment on why these villages have a higher incidence rate.

Study the incidence of neonatal tetanus in villages L to AA (where *no* cases were recorded in 1990). How many cases of neonatal tetanus occurred each year (1991–1994) in these villages compared with villages A to K? Comment on the difference observed; is it real, or is it perhaps the result of some statistical artefact?

Calculate the incidence rate per 1000 births in 1992, 1993 and 1994 for the two groups of villages, A to K and L to AA. Are the differences between the annual rates real or apparent?

In the light of this information about Jaya District, where would you expect cases of neonatal tetanus to occur in 1995? What action would you take with regard to this?

Exercise 73 (IV.3) Evaluating work progress

Objective: To be able to evaluate work progress.

Table III on page 386 represents the operational achievements for control of neonatal tetanus in the villages of Jaya District during 1991. It shows:

— the number of retrained TBAs
— the number of practising TBAs
— the percentage of practising TBAs who have been retrained
— the number of pregnant women who have been immunized
— the estimated total number of pregnant women
— immunization coverage of the district in terms of the percentage of pregnant women who have been immunized
— the number of messages diffused by village heads.

Assume that the 1991 targets were as follows:

— 20% of practising TBAs to be retrained
— 60% of pregnant women to be immunized
— 90% of village heads to have diffused 5 or more messages.

A. Calculate the percentage of retrained TBAs for the district as a whole and decide whether the retraining programme has achieved its target.

Table III. Operational outputs in the control of neonatal tetanus in Jaya District, 1991

Village	No. of retrained TBAs	No. of practising TBAs	Percentage of practising TBAs retrained	No. of pregnant women immunized	Estimated no. of pregnant women	Percentage of pregnant women immunized	Messages diffused by village chief
A	1	2	50	200	400	50	5
B	—	1	—	160	200	80	8
C	1	3	55	220	400	55	5
D	—	1	—	200	300	66	7
E	1	2	50	180	300	60	7
F	1	4	25	200	400	50	5
G	—	—	—	0	200	0	—
H	—	1	—	150	250	60	6
I	—	2	—	150	300	50	4
J	1	3	33	250	400	63	5
K	—	1	—	100	150	66	8
L	1	1	100	100	350	29	1
M	—	2	—	100	200	50	4
N	—	1	—	30	200	15	—
O	1	3	33	120	300	40	7
P	—	1	—	100	300	33	4
Q	—	2	—	30	200	15	4
R	—	1	—	80	100	80	6
S	1	1	100	100	400	25	—
T	—	1	—	100	250	40	3
U	1	2	50	160	200	80	5
V	—	1	—	30	200	15	5
W	—	1	—	100	300	33	2
X	—	2	—	90	200	45	4
Y	—	1	—	120	200	60	7
Z	—	1	—	130	250	52	5
AA	—	1	—	100	300	33	3
				Total: 3300	Total: 7250	Mean 46	

In how many individual villages has retraining been completed? In how many villages has retraining been started and in how many has it yet to start?

List the villages where immunization targets have been met. Using the data supplied in Exercise 72, compare immunization coverage with incidence of neonatal tetanus.

List the villages where communication targets have not been achieved; compare your findings with the data for incidence of tetanus. Calculate the percentages of villages in which 5 or more messages *have* been diffused.

B. Concentrate on villages E, J and U; what do they have in common? Is any other village in the same situation? How many villages would you have expected to meet similar targets in 1991? (*Hint*: assume that all 27 villages will be fully covered by 1995.)

C. Concentrate on villages B, D, H, K and Y; what common pattern do you find? How many cases of neonatal tetanus occurred in those villages in 1992 (refer to Table I in Exercise 72)? What common pattern can you find for villages A, C, F and O? How many cases of neonatal tetanus occurred in those villages in 1991 (again refer to Table I in Exercise 72)?

Comment on the results of the programme in these two groups of villages: are they different?

D. There are 14 villages in which no activity or only one activity reached the targets set. Identify them. How many cases of neonatal tetanus occurred in these villages in 1992?

Is this experience different from that in the two groups of villages in Part C of this exercise? Is it different from that in the villages considered in Part B?

E. Assume that the information in Tables I and II (Exercise 72) and Table III (opposite) are available to you to appraise the performance of two members of your staff, designated A and L. They are of equal seniority and have the same qualifications. Staff member A is responsible for the implementation of programmes in villages A to K, and staff member L has the same responsibility for villages L to AA.

Consider the target population in the two groups of villages and decide which staff member has the greater work-load. Then compare results and achievements in the two groups of villages for which these staff members are responsible:

	Staff member A Villages A–K	Staff member L Villages L–AA
Percentage of TBAs retrained Percentage of pregnant women immunized Number of messages diffused Number of villages reaching 2 or 3 targets		

On the basis of this comparison, comment on the performance of these two staff members.

Can you think of one factor — other than the work-loads of the two staff members — that might explain the different results and achievements in the two groups of villages?

F. Assume that the difference observed between targets and achievements is not a result of work-loads but of differences in the two staff members' abilities. Think of three areas in which differences in ability could explain differences in performance. Identify the steps you would follow in determining whether one particular ability actually accounted for the difference in performance.

> **NOW FILL IN**
> **THE EVALUATION SHEET**
> **THAT FOLLOWS**

Evaluation of Part IV

On the 0 to 5 scale, mark with a tick (✓) the extent of your agreement with the following statements:

Reading material is:

relevant to my work	0—/—/—/—/—/—5
useful for my work	0—/—/—/—/—/—5
difficult to understand	0—/—/—/—/—/—5
too time-consuming	0—/—/—/—/—/—5

Individual exercises are:

relevant to the subject	0—/—/—/—/—/—5
useful as means of learning	0—/—/—/—/—/—5
difficult to perform	0—/—/—/—/—/—5
too time-consuming	0—/—/—/—/—/—5

Group exercises are:

relevant to the team's work	0—/—/—/—/—/—5
useful for the team's work	0—/—/—/—/—/—5
difficult to perform	0—/—/—/—/—/—5
too time-consuming	0—/—/—/—/—/—5

I have acquired:

new knowledge	0—/—/—/—/—/—5
new attitudes	0—/—/—/—/—/—5
new skills	0—/—/—/—/—/—5

Possible solutions to exercises

Note: Only after careful individual preparation can well-managed group discussions reach 'correct' solutions to the exercises proposed. What follows is merely an illustration of some possible solutions suggested by the writers of the exercises.

Solution 1 (I.1) Management by objectives

Individual work

Reduce the incidence of poliomyelitis, measles and whooping cough.
Deliver 60% of babies under midwife's supervision.
Provide safe water at the rate of one pump per 20 households.
Conduct a family planning clinic at the health centre once a week.
Run a continuing-education programme for the staff of the health centre.

Such objectives help:

— in defining a work programme
— in assigning staff
— in assessing the effectiveness of services
— in assessing the efficiency of the team.

Group work

The first objective is a community health objective, the next two are service objectives, the third and fourth also define tasks which staff must perform, and the last refers to resources.

In such 'a hierarchy of objectives', each level supports the next higher level. In the case of objectives that are stated but not being pursued, means of achieving them should be designed and implemented, after finding out why this has not been done so far.

Solution 2 (I.1) Learning from experience

Individual work

"I learned from a discussion with a village chief how I could improve my immunization coverage."

Knowledge gained: a local tradition and belief.
Attitude change: to accept this belief and learn how to adapt to it.
Skill acquired: what to say to convince people and how to say it.
Relevance: immunization, specifically for diphtheria, tetanus and pertussis (DTP).
Evidence: my coverage increased from 40% in 1991 to 55% in 1992.

The programme supervisor was present at the meeting with the village chief, but I am not aware that anybody else heard about it. Perhaps it is important enough to discuss this in a staff meeting.

Group work

Performance is proof of competence.
Sharing experience would be a sound basis for developing the continuing-education programme.
Designing a formal exchange of knowledge, attitudes and skills should be assigned to competent staff at district level.

At the health centre, the public health nurse will implement the programme and direct meetings.

Solution 3 (I.1) Task analysis in team-work

Individual work

Activity: *Family Planning Clinic Consultation*					
Tasks \ **Name and designation**	**Myself Aisha, midwife**	**Other people helping with the work**			
		1) Ada, auxiliary midwife	**2) Sahib, doctor**	**3) Suliman, dispenser**	**4) Habib, clerk**
a) Keep room clean and orderly	✓	✓			
b) Patient registration and recording		✓			
c) History taking	✓				
d) Physical examination	✓		✓		
e) Health education — contraceptive methods	✓		✓		
f) Issue of contraceptives				✓	
g) Recording and appointment system		✓			✓
h) Notifying family planning programme officer	✓				
i) Keeping updated on family planning issues	✓	✓	✓		
j) Maintain stock of contraceptives			✓	✓	

Group work

Such analysis and assignment helps:

— in reminding us what needs to be done (work-plan)
— in coordinating our activities with those of other staff (duty roster)
— in finding out learning needs of staff (continuing education, in-service training)
— in supervision.

Additional information required: time spent and resources required. Perhaps management tasks should also be more clearly defined.

Solution 4 (I.1) Using resources efficiently

Individual work

Resources used:

1) working space and equipment
2) consumable supplies, drugs
3) petrol, oil, for transport
4) staff time
5) papers, forms, for information and communication
6) funds in cash.

Tasks	Resources used in performing these tasks					
	1) Work space	2) Supplies	3) Petrol	4) Staff time	5) Papers	6) Funds
a) Keep room clean and orderly	✓			✓		
b) Patient registration and recording				✓	✓	
c) History taking				✓	✓	
d) Physical examination	✓			✓		
e) Health education — contraceptive methods	✓	✓		✓	✓	
f) Issue of contraceptives		✓				
g) Recording and appointment system				✓	✓	
h) Notify family planning programme officer				✓	✓	
i) Keep updated on family planning issues				✓	✓	
j) Maintain stocks of contraceptives				✓	✓	

Group work

The possible consequences of a shortage of supplies — for example, condoms — are as follows:

— if there are no supplies, advice to patients can be theoretical only
— staff time is wasted
— patients are dissatisfied
— there will be unwanted pregnancies
— the cost-effectiveness of the family planning programme will decrease.

Possible remedial actions are:

— create a revolving fund for contraceptive supplies at the health centre
— replenish stocks of condoms when only two weeks' supplies remain.

Solution 5 (I.1) Assigning management tasks

Individual work

Management tasks	Who is responsible within the health team					People outside the team
	1) Midwife	2) Aux. nurse	3) Doctor	4) Dispenser	5) Clerk	
a) Planning objectives	✓		✓			District medical officer
b) Evaluation of skills	✓	✓	✓	✓		Pro-gramme officers
c) Assignment of tasks	✓		✓	✓		
d) Maintenance of stocks			✓	✓	✓	
e) Direct control of education programme			✓			District public health nurse
f) Supervision of the above			✓			District medical officer

Group work

Difficulties encountered by staff:

— not skilled in management
— no time to perform these tasks
— no forms available
— no incentives

Translated in correct management terms by the health team as: management has not been included explicitly in the work-plan.

Solution 6 (I.2) Rules for decision-making

Individual work

Types of decision to be made by a midwife:

1) home or hospital delivery
2) referral to maternity hospital (for high-risk case)
3) make a nurse-midwife responsible for all MCH records
4) when to replenish stocks
5) how much time should be spared for continuing education
6) when to take compensatory leave for overtime.

Whether decision was made or not on some occasion:

1) not made: lack of information about risk to mothers
2) not made: referral is not officially the midwife's responsibility
3) made
4) not made in time: no proper rule exists
5) impossible: no responsibility, authority, rules, norms
6) delayed: responsible officer absent, rule about midwife's rights unclear.

Group work

The most common reasons for decisions not being made or being untimely or inappropriate are:

— lack of written rules or norms
— authority not delegated during absences.

The suggested remedial actions are;

— clear statements of responsibility to be included in post description
— clear guidance on authority to be obtained from supervisor in staff meetings
— staff group to prepare a draft set of rules for submission to the district health officer
— a circular from the district health officer communicating the applicable norms
— an improved system of information in support of decisions.

Solution 7 (I.1) Relating resources, activities and results

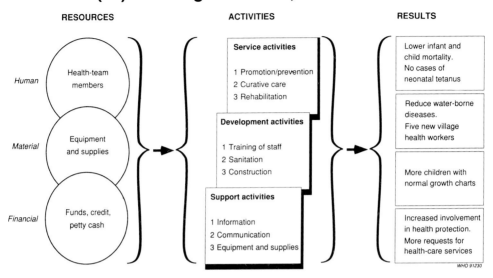

RESOURCES   ACTIVITIES   RESULTS

Human — Health-team members

Material — Equipment and supplies

Financial — Funds, credit, petty cash

Service activities
1 Promotion/prevention
2 Curative care
3 Rehabilitation

Development activities
1 Training of staff
2 Sanitation
3 Construction

Support activities
1 Information
2 Communication
3 Equipment and supplies

Lower infant and child mortality. No cases of neonatal tetanus

Reduce water-borne diseases. Five new village health workers

More children with normal growth charts

Increased involvement in health protection. More requests for health-care services

WHO 91230

Solution 8 (II.1) Know the community

Individual work

Information needed (opinions and beliefs)	How it may be obtained	Who should obtain it
1) Belief regarding illnesses which health service can help to cure	Survey in a sample of households	Public health nurse
2) Belief regarding illnesses which health service can help to prevent	Survey in a sample of households	Sanitarian
3) Belief regarding avoidable deaths	Group discussion with village health committee	Medical officer or medical assistant
4) Opinion on the suitability and effectiveness of health technology for 1), 2) and 3)	Questionnaire in follow-up of household survey	Village health committee
5) Opinion on the competence of health staff for 1), 2) and 3)	Questionnaire in follow-up of household survey	Village health committee
6) Opinion on the convenience of the services provided	Questionnaire in follow-up of household survey	Village health committee
7) Opinion on the personal relations between staff and clients	Household questionnaire	Village health committee
8) Belief/opinion as to who should make decisions on health matters in the household	Survey and group discussion	Medical officer Village health committee
9) Belief/opinion as to the role of a village health committee	'Complaint box' with village chairman	Medical officer Village chairman

Solution 9 (II.1) Understand the community

Individual or group work

Key people in the community:

Schoolmaster, headmaster, traditional chief, mayor, religious leaders, shopkeepers, health workers, members of the local council, social-development agents, representatives of official services, women's groups or non-governmental organizations.

Solution 10 (II.1) Discuss and decide

Individual work

Decisions needed about health programme	Methods and activities for reaching decisions	Most suitable people to participate
To agree on a village health programme	Village health committee meetings	Medical officer Medical assistant Village health committee
To conduct surveys	Consultations	Village chief Chairman of health committee Medical officer or assistant
To organize 'community sanitation weeks'	Public meetings	Sanitarians Village chief Village health committee
To establish a village pharmacy	Village health committee meetings	Public health nurse Village health committee
To adjust working hours of health centre to suit community needs	Health staff meetings	Medical officer or assistant Chairman of health committee Health centre staff

Solution 11 (II.1) Motivate and participate

Villagers' motivating factors	*Health workers' motivating factors*
Specific health needs perceived	Specific learning needs perceived
Desire to improve health status	Desire for promotion
Believe something can be done	Wish to get away from routine
Hope of personal benefit	Competition with colleagues
Will to be heard	Hope to enjoy learning
Feeling that they have something to offer	Feeling that their own capabilities are not being used
etc.	etc.

Villagers' demotivating factors

Non-perception of specific need
Negative past experiences
Fear of some negative effects of
programme
Fear that only some people will
derive benefit
Feeling of wasted effort
Inconvenient timing
etc.

Health workers' demotivating factors

Hard work in addition to existing
duties
Negative past experience of continuing-education programmes
Fear of added responsibilities
Fear of not succeeding as well as
colleagues
Not seeing opportunities to apply
acquired learning
Inconvenient timing
etc.

What health worker needs to do

Tell villagers about needs
Convince villagers of benefits of
programmes
Elicit villagers' objections and
suggestions
Encourage villagers' participation
Adjust programme to suit
villagers
Publicly commit health worker's
support
etc.

What health worker needs to learn

How to inform villagers
What to say about proposed pro-
gramme (purpose, methods, timing)
How to elicit expression of objec-
tions and suggestions
What are convincing arguments
How to enlist support
etc.

Solution 12 (II.1) Assess

Possible indicators of:

Communication

1) Proportion of villagers' perceived health problems known to health
   workers.
2) Proportion of health services provided known to villagers.
3) Number of complaints recorded in health centre.

Association

4) Number of decisions made (monthly)

   — by medical officer/medical assistant
   — by health team as a whole

— by village chief
— by village health committee
— by health team and committee together
— in public meetings.

5) Proportion of decisions made individually, and collectively.

Motivation

6) No personal contacts between health worker and heads of household.
7) List of demotivating factors mentioned by heads of households.
8) List of corresponding actions taken by health workers.

Participation

 9) Number of community members participating, by programme or service and location.
10) Number of persons served by health workers, by programme and location.
11) Proportion of those eligible who are served.

Who collects/processes indicators	*Where indicators are collected*
1) Medical officer or medical assistant	Supervision visits
2) Health workers	At health centre and in households
3) Medical officer or medical assistant	At staff meetings
4) Medical officer/medical assistant and health committee chairman	In coordination meetings
5) District health officer	In monthly reports
6) Health worker 7) Health worker 8) Health worker	In diary, reviewed in staff meetings, reported in monthly reports
9) Health worker responsible for programme 10) Health worker responsible for programme	Recorded on location, reviewed in supervision visits, discussed in staff meetings
11) Medical officer or medical assistant	Reported to district health officer

Solution 13 (II.1) Community participation

Because of the nature of this exercise no solution is indicated.

Solution 14 (II.2) Setting health-care objectives

Additional objectives of people may include:

P7) getting free services
P8) having equal access to services
P9) being safe from epidemics
P10) ensuring better survival of children.

Additional objectives of health authorities may include:

A7) delivering 2.5 services per person per year
A8) securing 6% of government budget
A9) applying higher technology in teaching institutions
A10) satisfying public demand.

Health workers' objectives may include:

W1) earning a living
W2) doing something useful
W3) helping suffering people
W4) reaching a desirable social status
W5) having security of employment
W6) doing an interesting job
W7) achieving promotion to higher responsibilities
W8) promoting scientific ideas
W9) performing a leadership role
W10) improving prospects for their own children.

Review of objectives of people and health authorities

Objectives P1, P2 — consistent with A1, A2
P3, P4 — *not* consistent with specific objectives except A6, A10
P5, P6 — consistent with A5, A6, A8, A10
P7, P8 — consistent with A3, A4

The people's objectives are consistent, but the health authorities' objectives A5 and A6 conflict with A8. Therefore:

— add specific objectives of health authorities to support P3, P4
— rewrite A10 explicitly to support equal accessibility and quality of service
— modify P7 to specify public *and* community funding as a basis for free service to individuals.

Review of health workers' objectives

The health workers' objectives do not contradict one another or those of the people or health authorities, *but* none of the health workers' objectives *explicitly* supports the objectives of the health authorities or the people's objective of equal accessibility and quality of free care. Therefore, rewrite the health workers' objectives W2, W3, W6 and W8 so that they explicitly support the provision of services and the quality of care. For instance:

W2 contributing to attainment of the health authorities' objectives A1 to A4
W3 helping achieve people's objectives P7 and P8.

Another of the health workers' objectives might perhaps be restated:

W7 updating knowledge, skills and experience to meet the expectations of the people and the health authorities, and thus to accede to higher responsibilities.

Solution 15 (II.2) Supervision

Individual work

A *good supervisor*:

— is fair with all
— issues clear instructions
— appreciates good work and initiative
— helps in overcoming staff difficulties
— does not accuse or criticize anyone in public.

All this helps health workers feel themselves to be partners in the job and to develop self-confidence.

A *poor supervisor*:

— consistently finds fault
— gives no praise
— does not communicate decisions to the interested parties
— is not helpful in developing workers' skills
— has 'favourites' among staff.

All this makes workers feel insecure and helpless, and does nothing to encourage initiative.

Conclusion: achievement of objectives depends on the supervisor's management skills and leadership role.

Solution 16 (II.2) Delegation

Individual work

A *medical officer* thinks about delegation:

1) "My job description says I am responsible for insertion of intrauterine devices as part of the family planning programme. I feel the midwife could do it just as well as I can."

2) "I am also responsible for the health education of the public, including patients. I feel that *all* staff should participate in health education."

Reasons:

1) "There are more than enough important tasks requiring my technical skill to keep me fully occupied."

2) "When it comes to communicating with the local people, my staff are better able than I am to make things understood."

Skills required:

1) "The midwife needs the skill to undertake IUD insertion, and good communication abilities. She must have high moral standards to perform that delicate function."

2) "All staff must know what the priority health problems are and what kinds of behaviour contribute to them. They must be able to communicate the necessary information to the public, simply and clearly. They must show a sympathetic attitude to patients and to the public."

A *staff member* thinks about delegation of

1) "coordination of all health education activities" (management task)
2) "preparation of written health education materials for village health workers" (support task)
3) "studying the impact of health education on patients' behaviour, and designing a set of questions or a checklist for assessing it" (learning task).

Reasons:

"I should welcome these assignments because they will improve:

— the use of my work time (more efficient health education materials)
— patients' chances of being cured and keeping well (through provision of better and more consistent information and advice)
— people's use of health services
— the use of precious resources (especially drugs)
— my own standing among colleagues and village health workers."

Authority necessary:

"I should be allowed to suggest changes in job descriptions, if necessary, to include more specific references to health education tasks.

I will need about 100 hours to produce the materials, to coordinate health education, and to assess its impact on patients' behaviour.

I must be authorized to organize the training of staff in methods of educating the public in health.

The District Health Officer should be involved in the delegation of such authority; I shall therefore submit drafts to the officer in charge of the health centre for his consideration and, after approval by the District Health Officer, to all staff of the health centre for information."

Drafts to be submitted:

— revised job description
— memo assigning authority
— circular to all staff of health centre.

Solution 17 (II.2) Resolving conflict

Group work

After discussion of the two case studies, a procedure should be agreed, to be observed by all staff and officers-in-charge in case of complaints and other situations leading to possible disciplinary action. The procedure should follow certain principles; for instance, all interested parties must be heard, witnesses must be interviewed, and a step-by-step process should be devised and recorded to include:

— verbal notification
— a written report
— interviews of those involved, separately and together
— staff meeting
— etc.

Solution 18 (II.2) Motivation

Some individuals will have more "agree" answers than "disagree"; others will have the opposite. It would be wise to discuss each statement in turn after scoring the individual answers. Discussion should be more thorough and searching where the scores are almost equally divided between "agree" and "disagree". The team should record what they agree upon for each statement.

Solution 19 (II.2) Self-evaluation of leadership

Because of the nature of this exercise no solution is indicated.

Solution 20 (II.2) Leadership and motivation

The completed table might look like the following:

Steps	Results	People		Timetable
		involved	**responsible**	
1) Review objectives of people, health authorities and health workers	See Exercise 14	Health team	MO or MA[a]	December
2) Record mutually supportive objectives	Agreed list of objectives		MO or MA	January
3) Identify needs and opportunities for delegation	See Exercise 16	Health team	MO or MA	January
4) Record agreed delegations	Agreed list of delegated tasks		MO or MA	February
5) Obtain authority to implement	Authorization of MO or MA	MO or MA	DHO[b]	March
6) Review the supervision function	See Exercise 15	Health team	MO or MA	March
7) Discuss motivation	See Exercises 18, 19	Health team	MO or MA	March
8) Prepare supervision schedule	Schedule		MO or MA	April
9) Draw up a conflict monitoring system	See Exercise 17	Selected health worker	MO or MA	May
10) Adopt a conflict monitoring system	Approved procedure	Health team	MO or MA	June
11) Assign arbitration powers in conflict resolution	Assignments	MO or MA	DHO	July

[a] MO = medical officer, MA = medical assistant.
[b] DHO = district health officer.

Solution 21 (II.3) Job description

Job title   Sanitarian (junior)

Job summary   Investigation of environmental health problems, delivery of environmental services, education of the public in sanitation matters and other measures for the promotion of environmental health, and control of environmental hazards in the district of assignment.

Duties	Preventive tasks, e.g. collection and forwarding of water samples, food samples, etc. Promotional tasks, e.g. advising and educating public on safe handling of food, safe disposal of excreta, etc. Control tasks, e.g. inspection of rubbish disposal sites, sanitary conditions of public institutions, etc. Supportive tasks, e.g. provision of chemicals to village health workers for water sterilization, rodent control, etc. Information tasks, e.g. collection, processing and diffusion of data on incidence of diarrhoea, household accidents, etc. Management tasks, e.g. planning, organizing and evaluating field visits. Learning tasks, e.g. maintaining awareness of need to improve skills or acquire new skills, looking for ways of learning such skills, reading environmental health journals, participating in continuing-education programme. Research tasks — as required by Provincial Environmental Health Officer.
Relations	To work under the technical supervision of the Provincial Environmental Health Officer and the administrative supervision of the District Medical Officer.
Training and development	Participation in in-service, on-the-job training and in continuing-education programmes. After six years of service the incumbent may apply for senior sanitarian posts.
Review and appraisal	Participation in two-weekly staff meeting with Environmental Health Officer to review activities and discuss problems. Annual written appraisal by, and interview with, superior, including opportunity to compare actual tasks with job description and to discuss performance and difficulties before appraisal is finalized and signed by both parties.

Solution 22 (II.3) Norms and standards

Objective	Safe water supply, storage and disposal in rural areas.

Related targets	One protected well within 500 metres of the houses of 60% of the population. A properly maintained water storage jar in 80% of houses. Properly maintained drainage ditches from 100% of houses to the nearest sandpit/sedimentation pond.
Target population and area	10 000 people, 1500 houses, 50 wells, in 80 villages and hamlets, over an area of 100 km^2.

Related tasks and norms

Inspection of wells	All wells 3 times a year = 3 wells a week = 5 hours a week
Collection of water samples	All wells and 35% of storage jars = 9 samples a week = 2 hours a week
Disinfection of wells	Approx. 33% of wells = 1 disinfection a week = 2 hours a week
Inspection and disinfestation of drainage ditches	All once a year as part of house inspection = 20 inspections a week = (probably) 5 disinfestations a week = 3 hours a week
Collection of diarrhoea statistics	As part of house inspection = 20 a week = 2 hours a week
Health education	As part of house inspection = (probably) 10 education/demonstration sessions a week = 4 hours a week
Reporting	Once a month = 2 hours a week
Related quality standards	*Escherichia coli* in less than 5% of water storage jars. *E. coli* in less than 5% of protected wells. Mosquito larvae in less than 10% of drainage ditches. Incidence of diarrhoea — less than 1 attack per person per year.

Solution 23 (II.3) Coordination

Activity		Responsible person	Resource persons
1		District health education officer	Medical officer, Chairman of village health committee
2		Chairman of village health committee	Medical officer
3	W	Sanitarian (health centre)	DHEO, MO[a], environmental health officer
	S	Sanitarian (health centre)	DHEO, MO, EHO[b]
	N	Public health nurse (health centre)	DHEO, MO, district public health nurse
	FH	Midwife (health centre)	DHEO, MO, district midwife
	I	MO (health centre)	DHEO, health team
4		DHEO	MO
5		MO	Chairman and members of village health committee
6		DHEO	MO
7	A	Chairman of village A health committee	Sanitarian, PHN, MW[c], MO
	B	Chairman of village B health committee	Sanitarian, PHN, MW, MO
	C	Chairman of village C health committee	Sanitarian, PHN, MW, MO
8		MO	DHEO, Chairman of village health committee

[a] DHEO = district health education officer, MO = medical officer.
[b] EHO = environmental health officer.
[c] PHN = public health nurse, MW = midwife.

Whose activities are to be coordinated?

Week	Activity	People
1	1	DHEO, Chairman of village health committee
5	3	DHEO, MO, District public health nurse
	5	DHEO, MO
10	8	MO, DHEO
15	7(C)	Chairman of village health committee, health team

What coordination mechanisms should be applied?

Week	Activity	Coordination mechanisms
1	1	Planning meeting at health centre
5	3, 5	Coordination meeting at health centre
		Correspondence with district officers
10	8	Person-to-person discussions
		Circulation of evaluation notes
		Review meeting to prepare evaluation report
15	7 (C)	Administrative arrangement with medical officer
		Preparatory meeting with village health committee

Solution 24 (II.3) Communication

Methods of communications

Oral:	person-to-person discussions, group discussions, meetings, etc.
Written:	notes, letters, circulars, reports, articles, etc.
Non-verbal:	intonation, gestures, facial expressions, drawings
Media:	audio (radio) visual (film strips, overhead projection), audiovisual (television, films)

Nature of messages

Technical:	information, instructions, appraisals, etc.
Administrative:	rules, regulations, incentives, sanctions, etc.
Personal:	sympathy, support, disapproval, etc.
Public relations:	opinions, polls, publicity, etc.
Decisions:	yes/no, stop/go, more/less, etc.

Senders/receivers

A district public health nurse sends written instructions to health-centre public health nurses.
An educational video clip on AIDS is shown to school students.
A coordination meeting allows all participants to communicate orally and non-verbally about technical and administrative issues, before decision-making.

Choice of effective communication methods

Message	Sender	Receiver	Method (no.)
Request for leave	Staff member	Supervisor	Letter (1)
Technical instruction	District public health nurse	Health centre nurses	Memo (2)
Administrative order	District health officer	Medical officers	Circular (3)
Sharing objectives	Director-general of health	Medical officers Chairman, village health committee	Group discussions (4)
Consulting specialist	Medical assistant	Specialist	Referral slip (5)
Coordination	Individual staff members	Entire team	Staff meeting (6)
Performance appraisal	Supervisor	Staff member	Discussion (7), then report (8)
Conveying sympathy	Staff	Patient	Gesture (9), words (10)
Appreciation of good work	Team leader	Individual staff	Supervision visit (11)
Punishing indiscipline	Director	Subordinate	Letter (1)
Advice on use of condom	Midwife	Married woman, etc.	Flannelgraph (12)

Solution 25 (II.3) Meetings

Decisions urgently needed might be:

×   Reorganization of patient flow in the outpatient clinic (Item VI of agenda).

××   Planning of district health education campaign (Item III).
      Contents of next year's continuing-education programme (Item V).
      Purchase of drugs to replenish village pharmacies (Item VI).

××× Disciplinary action against a negligent driver (Item II).

Proposed agenda

Staff meeting on 12-2-92, from 12.00 to 13.30 hours, at the health centre, outpatient consultation room. Chairman Mr X, sanitarian; secretary Mrs Y, midwife.

Item I: Reading and approval of last meeting's minutes (enclosed).
                                                              (5 min)

Item II: (to be introduced by medical officer or medical assistant)
             Review of complaints from staff that transport is frequently
             unavailable, though duly requisitioned for official duties.

Driver's explanation.
Motion in favour of disciplinary action from District
Health Officer.   (10 min)

Item III: (to be introduced by medical officer or medical assistant)
Review of the proposed district health education plan (draft
attached)
Assignment of responsibilities for preparing educational
materials.
Discussion of timing and administrative issues.   (15 min)

Item IV: (to be introduced by health centre dispenser)
Review of statements of stock-in-hand (attached).
Selection of fast-moving essential drugs for immediate
re-supply.
Assignment of responsibility for purchase and distribution.
(15 min)

Item V: (to be introduced by chairman)
Review of last year's continuing-education programme
Suggestions for educational objectives to be achieved in
coming year (from the floor).
Assignment of responsibilities for consolidating suggestions and submission to District Health Education Officer
(20 min)

Item VI: (to be introduced by public health nurse)
Review of staff and patients' complaints concerning wasted
time and disorderly queuing in waiting area.
Suggestions (from the floor) for improving patient flow and
speeding services.
Assignment of responsibility for documenting the proposed
reorganization of patient flow, including specific task
assignments to staff.   (20 min)

Item VII   Summary (by medical officer or medical assistant) of
decisions made in the meeting.   (5 min)

Solution 26 (II.3) Conducting a meeting I

Possible measures are:

1) Designate a neutral staff member to review with the medical officer the
   pros and cons of the situation.
2) Set a limit of three minutes' speaking time for *all* speakers.

3) State politely that the discussion of the topic is over.
4) Agree with the Secretary.
5) Discreetly draw the speaker to the topic under discussion.
6) Openly criticize the members' unpreparedness and postpone the discussion until the next meeting.

Solution 27 (II.3) Conducting a meeting II

Possible actions are:

1) Point out to the chairman that the meeting has *not* voted on the motion and propose that the vote be taken without further discussion or postponed until a later meeting.
2) Signal discreetly to the chairman that the member has been talking for x minutes.
3) Seek the medical officer or assistant's interpretation of the adopted motion, and record it accordingly.
4) Apologize to the chairman for the lack of written evidence, and request the medical officer's recollection of what the decision was.

Solution 28 (II.3) Conducting a meeting III

Because of the nature of this exercise no solution is indicated.

Solution 29 (II.3) Learning

The completed table might look like the following:

Situation no.	Health care	Health promotion	Support activities	Management	Training	Research
1)				×		
2)	⊗		⊗			
3)		⊠			×	
4)		⊠		×		
5)				×		
6)						×
7)					×	
8)	×					

Comments:

- In many areas no subsequent training was available.
- In others (marked ⊗) some further training took place, but I still feel I have not mastered the subject.
- On reading a technical journal relating to situation 8, I became aware of my inadequacies in the clinical management of diabetes.
- I now feel competent in the areas marked: ☒

Solution 30 (II.3) Training I

If I am in charge of coordinating programme activities, I need the following:

- Knowledge of:
  — purpose of coordination
  — methods of coordination
  — how to assess whether coordination works
  — motivating and demotivating factors
  i.e. general management theory.

- Attitudes:
  — commitment to efficiency
  — sharing objectives with others
  — willingness to learn from mistakes
  — enthusiasm for inspiring commitment in others
  i.e. leadership qualities.

- Skills:
  — analysing work and results
  — scheduling activities
  — assigning responsibilities
  — monitoring work progress
  i.e. practical dispositions and application.

I shall also need the authority to coordinate the activities.

Ways of learning:

- To acquire basic knowledge:
  — reading
  — experience-sharing
  — seminars
  — learning by doing.

- To develop attitudes:
  — learning by doing
  — workshops
  — role-play
  — experience-sharing.

- To improve skills:
  — workshops
  — learning by doing
  — experience-sharing
  — reading.

To learn how to coordinate programme activities I suggest, over the coming 12 weeks:

1) A group discussion (in a staff meeting) to review and share acquired experiences (K, A, S).
2) A management seminar to acquire basic principles and concepts (K), followed by recommended reading.
3) A workshop with practical exercises on coordination (K, A, S).
4) A period of learning-by-doing, followed by an assessment (A, S).
5) A group discussion (in a staff meeting) to review progress, and discuss difficulties needing resolution (K, A, S).

I, myself, would be primarily concerned with this learning process, but I think that all those whose activities I am expected to coordinate should take part in all the steps 1–5.

After completion, the proposed programme of in-service learning activities on the topic "organizing supervision" may look like the following:

Learning activity	People responsible	participating	Date and place	
Group discussion on supervision	MO or MA[a]	Health team	30/8	Health centre
Seminar on community health problems and objectives, service targets and norms of perform-ance	District health officer	MO/MA Health team	9/9	District headquarters
Reading on evaluation methods and of past activity reports	MO or MA	Health team	1/9 to 30/9	Health centre
Role-play on how to guide, support and encourage through supervision	Visiting teacher	MO/MA Health team	1/10	Health centre
Group discussion on effectiveness, efficiency and economy	A district field supervisor	MO/MA Health team	15/10	Health centre
Workshop on checklists and schedules for supervision	District health officer	MO/MA Health team	30/10	Health centre
Field practice	MO or MA	Health team	1/11 to 30/12	Field
Group discussion on work progress	MO or MA	Health team	2/1	Health centre

[a] MO = medical officer, MA = medical assistant.

Solution 32 (II.4) Monitoring of performance

Health worker's measurement of own work performance:

number of outpatients seen   ×
number of new patients
number of repeat (follow-up) visits
number of home visits   ×
number of work hours   ×

The patient or client will be concerned more with:

waiting time
consultation time
quality of care
result of care
quality of personal relations
availability of drugs etc.   ×

The supervisor may be interested in:

worker's punctuality
volume of work done
technical skill of worker   ×
management skill of worker
communication skill
quality of records   ×
maintenance of equipment
consumption of supplies.

Others — for instance, the village health committee — may be concerned more with the health worker's:

dependability
accountability
sense of responsibility.

Solution 33 (II.4) Assessment of performance

The District Public Health Nurse assessed the following points during her supervision visit to an outpatient session:

Technical skills

1) completeness of history-taking
2) injection technique
3) maintenance of sterile equipment
4) content of health education etc.

Management skills

5) timing of patient flow
6) orderly arrangement of work space
7) record-keeping (notes on patients)
8) maintenance of stocks of disposable supplies
    etc.

Communication skills

 9) listening to patients
10) responding to patient's needs
11) quality of explanations given to patients
12) quality of working relations with other staff etc.

Faults found were summarized as follows:

Shortcomings observed	*Relevant norms/standards*
3) Poor maintenance of sterile equipment	Covered in "Nursing Manual"
4) Irrelevant information given to patients	Covered in "Nursing Manual"
7) Inadequate record-keeping	No descriptive norm available
8) Shortage of basic supplies	Covered in "Work Instructions"
10) No expression of sympathy	General guidance only
12) Shouting at room attendant	No guidance available

Factors contributing to the shortcomings were as follows:

Importance

Processes:
   3) insufficient day-to-day *supervision* by medical officer/medical assistant in charge
   4) inadequate *training* in health education (in continuing-education programme)   3
   7) responsibilities for record-keeping not clearly assigned
   8) no *monitoring* of stock to allow timely replenishment
  11) poor *coordination* of work in outpatient area   2

Resources:
   4) no health education *documentation* available
   7) no filing cabinet or box for keeping *records*   4
   8) certain items *unavailable* from central stores

Personal:
   3) medical officer *not interested* in staff problems and health worker *does not like* to ask help or clarification
  10) health worker has a *sick child* at home and did not pay attention to patient's needs   1
  12) health worker scolded the room attendant who seems never to *understand or follow instructions*.

To improve the situation:

— help staff solve the problem of sick children
— organize more systematic day-to-day supervision
— arrange staff meetings to solve problems of work organization
— review continuing-education needs and organize training
— discuss information issues (patients' records, stock monitoring) and assign responsibilities clearly
— treat staff conflict seriously.

Solution 34 (II.4) Control

Individual work

The following are suggestions for corrective action:

— observation of shortcomings in staff performance
— discussion with concerned staff on observed shortcomings
— help in resolving personal problems, family crises, etc.
— generate renewed staff interest in the job
— participation in staff activities, e.g. staff meetings to resolve organizational difficulties and staff training for needed skills
— mediation in and solution of staff conflict
— better use of resources and better information.

Group work

Action	Decision-maker	Responsible persons	Obstacles	Time-frame	Cost
Supervise	MO or MA and/or DHO[a]	Health staff (may specify what is expected of supervisor)	Too little time given to supervision	Should be possible over next 3 months	None, except in time
Staff coordination (meetings)	MO or MA	Health staff (must specify issues)	No suitable place for meetings	Once weekly, with immediate effect	None, except in staff time
Continuing education and training	DHO	Health staff (must determine needs)	Insufficient skills and documontation	One hour every afternoon	Cost of documentation
Conflict resolution procedure	MO or MA	Health staff (must report conflicts)	Hidden sources of personnel conflict	As required, with immediate effect	None

[a] MO = medical officer, MA = medical assistant, DHO = district health officer.

Solution 35 (II.4) Records and reports

Information required for monitoring and assessing performance (*observed* data):

		Available
working hours, of staff:	40 hours weekly	×
work schedule, of staff:	duty record (assign-ments)	×
outpatient work, by programe by staff:	immunization home visits, consulta-tions, etc.	
use of work time:	technical activities (50%), management (20%), idle time (30%)	
resources used, by programme: by staff:	biologicals (doses) petrol (and distance travelled), drug issues doses, cost)	×
frequency of complaints:	about waiting time, rude-ness	
population coverage, by programme: by staff:	numbers eligible, by age, sex and place numbers provided with services, by age, sex and place	×

etc.

Targets, norms and standards for the above, for comparison (assessment) of *observed* achievements with desired levels of performance:

	Available
— official working hours of health centre and staff	×
— weekly assignments of staff to various programmes, and/or night-duty rosters, etc.	
— programme targets, population eligible for various services	
— expected work output (norms), and standards of quality of care, for individual staff members	×
— expected time allocation, in each staff category, for services (preventive, curative, promotional), management functions, information processing (records, reports, filing), supportive tasks (sterilization, etc.), learning activities, staff meetings, meals and rest-breaks	×

— amounts of various resources expected to be available,
by programmes and by staff (based on budget and
other sources)
— acceptable complaint frequency (e.g. less than one
complaint per 1000 services delivered)
— etc.

To eliminate gaps between observation data and normative information, particularly with regard to the use and allocation of work time by function:

— specify targets, norms and standards, so that all staff understand their individual expected work-loads
— review and revise assignments to enable staff to undertake their expected service work-load
— allocate time clearly to the various functions involved in delivering services
— monitor the use of work time by staff, to permit rational discussion of performance
— assign responsibilities for monitoring and assessment, especially for recording and reporting
— feed back the available information into supervision and coordination mechanisms, to ensure continuous improvement of performance.

Solution 36 (II.4) Supervision

The following points may be covered as part of a supervisory visit:

— what staff can do (staff competence)
— what staff actually do (achievements)
— how staff perform (attitudes)
— what staff cannot do (difficulties, shortcomings) and why
— what staff should do (suggestions)
— what staff feel (personal problems, conflicts)
— what the patients feel.

In more detail, supervision should include a review of:

— objectives, targets and norms of performance (are they known, shared?)
— job descriptions, work instructions, duty rosters (do they exist, are they followed?)
— technical skills (have they been mastered, are they applied?)
— output of work, quality of care (do they meet targets and norms?)
— use of time (is it as scheduled, is it balanced?)

— communications skills with patients and other staff (is it effective or is it confrontational?)
— management skills (are there process or resource difficulties?)
— personal problems
— learning needs with regard to improvement of skills
— suggestions for remedying observed shortcomings, deficiencies and problems
— patients' appreciation of services (quality, quantity, timing, public relations).

The following are needed to make a supervisory visit successful:

— agenda prepared by supervisor and made known to staff
— preparation of relevant information
— sufficient time for supervisor to observe and talk to individuals
— meetings to discuss suggestions and finalize future programmes.

Solution 37 (III.1) Inventory of equipment

Health worker: Medical assistant   *Room*: Consultation room

Item	E/NE	Quantity available	State of repair			
			s	u	r	m
Table	NE	1	s			
Chairs	NE	2	1s		1r	
Weighing scale	NE	1		u		
Sphygmomanometer	NE	1	s			
Clinical thermometers		3	2s	1u		
Tongue depressors, metal	NE	2	s			
Scissors	NE	3	s			
Forceps	NE	1	(not known)			m
Clinical record cards	E	500	(not appl.)			m
Filing boxes for cards	NE	2	2s			
Gauze packs, sterile, 5, 10, 15 cm	E	2 packs each	s			
Steel box for gauze packs	NE	1	s			
Cotton, not sterile	E	500 g	s			
Steel box for cotton	NE	1	s			
Soap, liquid	E	500 ml	s			
Soap dispenser, metal	NE	1	s			
Ethanol	E	250 ml	s			
Ethanol container, glass	NE	1	s			
Disinfectant liquid	E	500 ml	s			
Container for disinfectant, glass	NE	1	s			
Syringes, disposable	E	22	s			
Needles, disposable	E	108	s			

Note: Drugs are *not* considered here.

Solution 38 (III.1) Requisition of supplies

Because all catalogues differ, no solution is indicated.

Solution 39 (III.1) Storage of expendables

A suggested storage cabinet might look like the following:

A Cotton, gauze Metal items	B Liquids and glassware	C Disposables Soap and detergent	D Office supplies
A1 Rags	B1 Methanol	C1 Syringes C2 Needles	D1 Record cards
A2 Gauze	B2 Ethanol	C3 Tongue depressors C4 Test-tubes, swabsticks	D2 Paper and envelopes
A3 Cotton	B3 Stains	C5 Soap (solid)	D3 Pens D4 Pencils D5 Erasers
A4 Adhesive tape	B4 Disinfectant fluids	C6 Detergents (solid)	D6 (empty)
A5 Metal boxes	B5 Glass ware	C7 (empty)	D7 (empty)

WHO 91231

Solution 40 (III.I) Keeping a stock ledger

The completed stock ledger for the period 1.4.93 to 1.5.93 should look like the following (where each line of the table represents a separate page of the ledger):

(Page no. in stock ledger)	Item	Date	Received from	Invoice no.	Quantity received	Quantity issued	Balance in stock
10	Cotton (absorbent)	1/4 14/4 1/5				2 kg	5 kg 3 kg 3 kg
14	Disinfectant	1/4 14/4 20/4 1/5	GMS[a]	497	2 litres	2 litres	3 litres 1 litre 3 litres 3 litres
18	Gauze	1/4 14/4 1/5				4 kg	8 kg 4 kg 4 kg
49	Needles (reusable)	1/4 14/4 1/5				200	2000 1800 1800
61	Record cards	1/4 14/4 1/5				800	5000 4200 4200
68	Soap (solid)	1/4 14/4 20/4 1/5	GMS	497	4 kg	2.4 kg	6 kg 3.6 kg 7.6 kg 7.6 kg
70	Syringes, 2 ml (reusable)	1/4 14/4 20/4 1/5	GMS	497	100	200	2000 1800 1900 1900
75	Test-tubes	1/4 20/4 1/5	GMS	497	200		1000 1200 1200
87	Methanol	1/4 14/4 1/5				4 litres	20 litres 16 litres 16 litres

[a] GMS = government medical stores.

Solution 41 (III.1) Maintenance and repair

Review of the consultation room and inventory (see Exercise 37) shows the following to be necessary:

Floor	needs cleaning
Walls	need whitewashing
Storage cabinet	needs orderly rearrangement
Table	needs cleaning
Chair (one)	needs repairing or replacing
Weighing scale	needs replacing
Forceps	needs finding

Staff responsible for requesting, authorizing and undertaking these tasks are as follows:

Action	Requesting	Authorizing	Undertaking
Cleaning	Health staff	Health staff	Health staff
Whitewashing	Staff/medical officer	District health officer	Contractor
Rearranging	Staff/medical officer	Staff	Staff
Repairing	Medical officer	District health officer	Contractor
Replacing	Medical officer	District health officer	Central medical stores
Finding	Medical officer	Staff	Staff

Solution 42 (III.2) Standard drug list

Drugs selected for a village health worker to dispense should be:

— safe in the hands of the health worker
— effective against specific conditions
— capable of curing or relieving most common conditions
— acceptable to the population (non-toxic)
— the cheapest that meet required standards of safety and effectiveness
— manufactured in the country, whenever possible.

The expected number of consultations at each one-day clinic might be as follows:

30 — adult men
50 — women of childbearing age
12 — pregnant women
12 — infants
26 — children aged 1 to 4 years

Then the estimated drug requirement for each one-day clinic would be as follows:

iron sulfate	for pregnant women	$30 \times 12 = 360$ doses
contraceptives	for women of child-bearing age	1 cycle $\times 50 = 50$ cycles
tetanus toxoid	for children and pregnant women	38 doses
vitamins	for pregnant women	$30 \times 12 = 360$ doses
protein supplement		
vaccines	for infants and pregnant women	38 doses
aspirin	for adult men and women	$5 \times 42 = 210$ doses
penicillin	for 10% of all patients	$5 \times 13 = 65$ doses
sulfadimidine	for 10% of all patients	$5 \times 13 = 65$ doses

Solution 43 (III.2) Stocking drugs

The standard drugs available in the health centre might be grouped as follows:

Analgesics and antipyretics (AA)

aspirin
paracetamol
phenobarbital

Antibacterials (AB)

procaine benzylpenicillin
sulfamethoxazole + trimethoprim
tetracycline
isoniazid

Cardiovascular (C)

digoxin
propranolol

Gastrointestinal (GI)

aluminium hydroxide
charcoal
piperazine
mebendazole

Genito-urinary system (GU)

diuretics
ergometrine

Respiratory tract (R)

cough mixture
ephedrine
aminophylline
codeine phosphate

Skin and eye (S)

benzoic acid
tincture of iodine
bacitracin ointment
tetracycline ointment

Vitamins and food supplements (VS)

retinol
ADEK supplement
iron sulfate

Sera, antitoxins and vaccines (SAV)

tetanus antitoxin ⎫
BCG vaccine ⎬ all to be stored in refrigerator
DPT vaccine ⎭

Dangerous drugs (DD)

morphine ⎫
pethidine ⎪
digoxin ⎬ all to be kept under lock and key
ergometrine ⎪
phenobarbital ⎭

Life-saving/emergency drugs (E)

chloroquine
quinine injection
benzylpenicillin
ergometrine injection
oral rehydration salts   } there must be permanent easy access to these
charcoal   drugs
ephedrine injection
epinephrine injection
chlorpromazine

A suitable storage system, based on the 'A/B' system, is illustrated below:

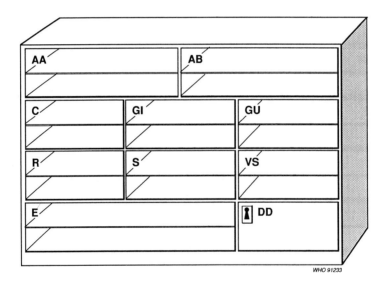

WHO 91233

Solution 44 (III.2) Monitoring a drug stock-card system

To improve the system, it would be valuable to introduce signed vouchers to show receipts of supplies in each department supplied by the central medical stores. For supervision of the system there should be regular monitoring of drugs supplied to each department.

Item: TETRACYCLINE (500 mg tablets)					
Date	From or to:	Received	Issued	Balance	Remarks
31/3/93				7 500	
1/4/93	CMS[a] (Invoice 612)	2 500		10 000	Expiry: Apr 1994 verified by MO[b]
2/4/93	Outpatients		1 200	8 800	
	Surgical ward		2 400	6 400	
15/4/93	Health centre 1		600	5 800	
	Health centre 2		700	5 100	
31/4/93				5 100	
1/5/93	CMS (Invoice 613)	2 500		7 600	Expiry: July 1994 verified by MO

[a] CMS = central medical stores.
[b] MO = medical officer.

Solution 45 (III.2) Monitoring drug use

The mean monthly consumption of a drug is the sum of the quantities of that drug issued over a stated period divided by the number of months in that period.

The proportion issued out of the latest stock in hand is the quantity of a drug issued between two delivery consignments divided by the quantity in stock after the second of the two deliveries. For instance, in Exercise 44, the proportion of tetracycline issued out of the latest stock in hand is 4900/7600 = 65% (which is rather high).

The information gleaned from stock cards for antibacterial drugs might be summarized as follows:

Drug	Date when out of stock	Consumption between consignments	Mean monthly consumption 1993	Proportion issued out of stock in hand
Procaine benzyl-penicillin (vials)	—	9 900	10 000	Approx. 45%
Sulfamethoxazole + trimethoprim (tablets)	16/4/93	17 500	15 000	>75%
Tetracycline (tablets)	—	4 900	5 000	Approx. 65%
Isoniazid (tablets)	—	8 600	8 000	Approx. 50%

Comments

In this group of groups only sufamethoxazole + trimethoprim tables ran out of stock. The consumption in April was higher than the mean monthly consumption and the proportion issued out of stock in hand was much higher than for most other drugs in the group.

The stock-card for sufamethoxazole + trimethoprim might look like the following:

Item: SULFAMETHOXAZOLE + TRIMETHOPRIM (1000 mg tablets)					
Date	**From or to:**	**Received**	**Issued**	**Balance**	**Remarks**
31/12/92				10 000	
1/1/93	CMS[a] (Invoice 609)	12 000		22 000	Expiry: Apr 1994 verified by MO[b]
31/1/93	Patients		16 000	6 000	
1/2/93	CMS (Invoice 610)	12 000		18 000	Raise requisition to 15 000 (signed by MO)
28/2/93	Patients		14 000	4 000	
1/3/93	CMS (Invoice 611)	12 000		16 000	
31/3/93	Patients		15 000	1 000	
1/4/93	CMS (Invoice 612)	12 000		13 000	
Up to 16/4/93	Patients		13 000		

[a]CMS = central medical stores.
[b]MO = medical officer.

Comments

From early 1993, monthly issues exceeded monthly receipts. By monitoring "proportion issued out of stock in hand", a shortage could have been anticipated: the proportion was 73% in January, 77% in February, and 90% in March, but should have been below 50% to maintain an adequate monthly reserve. Despite the medical officer's decision in February to raise the monthly requisition to 15 000, consignments were still limited to 12 000 up to April. Stock in hand therefore fell from 10 000 at the end of December 1992 to 1000 at the end of March 1993. Moreover, consumption in the first half of April was almost equal to the previous mean monthly consumption (because of an epidemic). Assuming a subsequent return to normal consumption (7500 tablets per half-month, treatment courses of 5 days × 2 tablets daily), as many as 750 patients may be denied treatment in the second half of April as a result of the shortage.

Solution 46 (III.2) Preparing a drug requisition

The stock card for sulfamethoxazole + trimethoprim revealed that the drug being used is Bactrim, a brand-name preparation costing 10 monetary units (MU) per 1-gram tablet. The corresponding generic preparation, available internationally, costs only 4 MU per 1-gram tablet.

If the generic preparation were requisitioned rather than the brand-name product, monthly expenditure of 120 000 MU would represent 30 000 tablets of generic drug instead of 12 000 tablets of Bactrim. In that case the monthly consumption (15 000) could be covered, and the "proportion issued out of latest stock in hand" could be kept below 50%, thus ensuring a full month's reserve.

Moreover, after rebuilding the stocks to a reasonable level, the expenditure on this drug could be reduced without inconvenience to patients.

Solution 47 (III.2) Analysing drug prescriptions

Prescription No.	Drug name and group		BN/GD	Unit	Amount prescribed
1	paracetamol	AA	GD	pill	15
	ADEK supplement	VS	GD	pill	30
2	procaine penicillin	AB	BN	vial	5
	cough mixture	R	GD	ml	150
3	charcoal	GI	GD	pill	20
	ADEK supplement	VS	GD	pill	30
4	benzoic acid	S	GD	ml	100
5	phenobarbital	AA	GD	pill	30
	iron sulfate	VS	GD	pill	100
	ADEK supplement	VS	GD	pill	30
6	sulfadimidine	AB	GD	pill	10
	codeine sulfate	R	GD	ml	150
	paracetamol	AA	GD	pill	10
7	bacitracin ointment	S	BN	ml	10
8	piperazine	GI	GD	ml	150
9	aspirin	AA	GD	pill	10
	sulfadimidine	AB	BN	pill	20
	aluminium hydroxide	GI	GD	ml	150
	ADEK supplement	VS	GD	pill	30
10	streptomycin	AB	GD	vial	30
	isoniazid	AB	GD	pill	300
	codeine sulfate	R	BN	ml	150

Number of drugs prescribed:	22						
Number of prescriptions with	1	2	3	4	5	6+	drugs
no.	3	3	3	1	—	—	

Most commonly prescribed drug:	ADEK supplement (prescribed four times)

Number of prescriptions for drugs of group:	AA	AB	C	GI	GU	R	S	VS	SAV	DD
no.	4	5	—	3	—	3	2	5	—	—

Proportion of brand-name drugs prescribed $= 4/22 = 18\%$

Comments

All the 'fast-moving' drugs prescribed are generic except those in the AB group. Savings could be made by reducing the frequency of prescription of ADEK vitamin supplements, and by prescribing reliable generic antibacterials instead of brand-name products. This would allow more essential, fast-moving generic drugs to be requisitioned.

'Slow-moving' drugs are those in the C, GU, and DD groups; from a review of stock cards, it appears that none of these drugs has an expiry date before the end of 1993. Delay in reordering these drugs for some time will lead to savings, without immediate risk of running short.

Amounts prescribed:	
in the AA group:	average prescribed $= 50 \div 5 = 10$ doses (or days)
in the AB group:	prescriptions cover in *one* case: 30 days (for tuberculosis) otherwise: $35 \div 3 = 11$ doses (or days)
in the VS group:	average prescribed: $220 \div 5 = 44$ doses (or days)
in the other groups:	prescriptions cover $50 \div 6 = 6$ days on the average.

Comment

Vitamin supplements and AA and AB drugs (except antituberculosis) could be prescribed for one week at a time, thus reducing probable wastage. The likely 30–40% saving that would result might solve part of the 'fast-moving' drugs problem.

Solution 48 (III.2) Assessing patients' use of drugs

Patients' answers to the questions might be as follows:

1) Seven out of ten patients had heard about the prescribed treatment, five from other patients and two from health workers.
2) Six out of ten patients trusted the efficacy of the treatment; the other four patients didn't know.
3) One patient of the ten feared side-effects from the treatment, claiming to have a 'weak stomach'.
4) Four of the ten patients would have preferred a different treatment; one gave no reason for the preference and three wanted injections.
5) Nine out of ten patients confirmed that they intended to complete the course of treatment.
6) Nine out of ten patients knew how many drugs they were supposed to take in the course of their treatment, eight of the ten knew how many pills this involved, six knew how many times a day each drug should be taken, and five were aware of how many days the treatment lasted.

At the second interview, patients' answers might be as follows:

7) Three patients said their condition had not improved at all, two said there had been a little improvement, four said they were much better and one very much better.
8) Of the eight patients who took the full course of treatment, three were from the groups claiming little or no improvement and five from the groups claiming to be much or very much improved.
9) Of four patients who expressed a wish to continue the treatment or to have different treatment, two were from the groups claiming little or no improvement in their condition and two from the groups claiming to be much or very much improved.

Comparisons

Five improved patients said "yes" to questions 1 and 2. They included one who feared side-effects of the treatment and two who would have preferred a different treatment. All five patients understood how to take the treatment and stated that they intended to take it.

Of the five patients who said they felt little or no improvement, four said they did not trust the treatment but intended to take it anyway. Two would have preferred a different treatment. None could say fully how the treatment should be taken, but three said they had taken the full course. Two wished for further treatment.

Solution 49 (III.3) Maintaining accounts I (allocation ledger)

Equipment/supplies/services	Allocation (annual)
Drug supplies	1000 MU[a]
Office equipment	100 MU
Staff transport	250 MU
Printing of education materials	100 MU
Car, petty repairs and maintenance	500 MU

[a] MU = monetary units.

The ledger page pertaining to minor repairs and maintenance of the car may look as follows:

Date	Description/Purpose	Document reference (folio no.)	Order or requisition (debit)	Allocation (credit)
1/1/93	Annual allocation	Notification Memo no. 65 dated 31/12/92		500 MU
17/4/93	Recharging of battery	Bill no. 91/1 dated 30/4/93 Voucher no. 88 certified on 1/5/93	4.50 MU	495.50 MU
3/5/93	Repair of punctured tyre	Bill no. 91/7 dated 30/5/93 Voucher no. 104 certified on 1/6/93	3.50 MU	492 MU
2/7/93	Repair of speedometer gauge, replacement of cable	Bill no. 91/15 dated 20/7/93 Voucher no. 132 certified on 1/8/93	29.5 MU	462.50 MU
21/9/93	Replacement of windshield	Accident report dated 30/8/93 Estimates dated 5/9, 6/9, 7/9/93 Bill no. 91/32 Voucher no. 174 certified on 30/9/93	172 MU	290.50 MU

Solution 50 (III. 3) Maintaining accounts II (petty-cash book)

Items that may be paid for out of petty cash include:

— postage stamps
— electricity charges
— bus fares for official duties
— supplies for maintenance of health centre
   etc.

For these purposes, petty cash is provided to

— medical officer
— health centre clerk
— administrative assistant
— other staff members (health visitors, sanitarians, etc.).

A single imprest account is maintained by the medical officer, with sub-imprest accounts maintained by the staff concerned:

— clerk has a 20 MU (monetary units) sub-imprest
— health visitor has a 10 MU sub-imprest
— sanitarian has a 10 MU sub-imprest
— administrative assistant has a 50 MU sub-imprest.

The total imprest amount available to the medical officer is 150 MU.

Each staff-member provided with sub-imprest money maintains a petty-cash book as shown on page 193. The medical officer's imprest account book may appear as shown on page 194.

To get the imprest replenished, each staff member must show the original receipts for money spent to the medical officer.

Solution 51 (III.4) Managing time: self-assessment

Auxiliary nurse's use of time (summary):

Tasks	Start time	Finish time	Time used (min)
Receiving and registering out-patients and taking and recording case histories of new patients	07.30	09.00	90
Assisting medical officer and instructing and explaining to patients (and parents)	09.00	12.00	180
Tea/lunch-breaks	12.00	13.00	60
Staff meeting	13.00	14.00	60
Assisting with MCH clinic and health education of mothers	14.00	16.00	120
Sterilizing instruments and putting health education materials away	16.00	16.30	30
Unaccounted for (non-productive time)			25
Total work time			480 = 8 h

Solution 52 (III.4) Observing use of time

Registration and interviewing of patients/parents

Time for each patient: (1) 3.5 min (2) 2.5 min (3) 5 min (4) 3 min (5) 1.5 min (6) 4 min (7) 3.5 min . . . . (19) 2.5 min (20) 3 min.

Number of patients observed: 20
Mean time per patient: 3 minutes
Total number of patients registered: 27
Total time for patient registration: $27 \times 3 = 81$ minutes.

Assisting medical officer in consultation (introducing patient, summarizing case history, preparing patient, recording clinical observations, preparing and giving injections, etc.)

Time for each patient: (1) 5 min (2) 4 min (3) 6 min (4) 3 min (5) 2.5 min (6) 4.5 min (7) 8 min (8) 3.5 min (9) 4 min (10) 5 min.

Number of patients observed: 10
Mean time per patient: 4.5 minutes
Total number of patients examined: 27
Total time for assisting medical officer: $27 \times 4.5 = 122$ minutes

Instructing and advising patients (explaining treatment and need for return visits, etc., advising on diet and hygiene).

Time for each patient: (1) 1 min (2) 2 min (3) 2 min (4) 1.5 min (5) 1 min (6) 1 min (7) 2 min (8) 1 min (9) 1.5 min (10) 1.5 min (11) 2 min (12) 1.5 min.

Number of patients observed: 12
Mean time per patient: 1.5 minutes
Total number of patients advised: 27
Total time for instruction of patients: $27 \times 1.5 = 40$ minutes.

Supportive tasks (sterilizing equipment, filing records, etc.)

Between 15.45 and 16.30:
   sterilizing: 16 minutes
   filing: 25 minutes

Total time for support tasks: 41 minutes (i.e. $41/27 = 1\frac{1}{2}$ minutes per patient).

Staff meeting (technical and administrative topics)

Duration: 30 minutes (from 13.00 to 13.30)

Non-productive use of time

07.30–08.00	Unproductive time in consulting room	20 min
09.45–10.00	Tea-break	15 min (10 allowed)
11.50–12.00	Telephone call	10 min
12.00–13.15	Lunch-break	75 min (45 allowed)
16.00–17.00	Unproductive time in consulting room	7 min
16.10–16.20	Tea-break	10 min (10 allowed)
	Total unproductive time	137 min (65 allowed)

Unproductive time as a proportion of the working day: $(137-65)/480$
$$= 15\%$$

Comments

Use of time for patient-oriented tasks is not balanced — 3 minutes for registration and case histories and 4.5 minutes for assisting with consultations compared with only 1.5 minutes for health education. Less time should be spent assisting with consultations and more should be devoted to health education. However, adding in the 2 minutes per patient spent on support tasks, a total of 11 minutes per patient is satisfactory.

Unproductive time, other than that which is allowed, should be made available for useful activities, such as learning.

Solution 53 (III.4) Assessing allocation of time by function

Use of Public Health Nurse's time by function:

Function	Day						Total time
	1	2	3	4	5	6	
Preventive care	—	220 min	25 min	180 min	30 min	—	7 h 35 min
Curative care	155 min	50 min	140 min	30 min	120 min	—	8 h 15 min
Health promotion	60 min	90 min	50 min	90 min	60 min	—	5 h 50 min
Supportive tasks	95 min	30 min	80 min	50 min	30 min	—	4 h 45 min
Management	30 min	30 min	50 min	45 min	40 min	30 min	3 h 45 min
Information	20 min	40 min	35 min	45 min	50 min	20 min	2 h 30 min
Learning	30 min	30 min	20 min	15 min	20 min	180 min	4 h 55 min
Research	—	30 min	10 min	25 min	—	10 min	1 h 15 min
Main duty area for the day	Out-patients	MCH field visits	Out-patients	School health service	Out-patients	Staff develop-ment	*Total* 38 h 50 min

Total work time accounted for, 38 h 50 min, represents 97% of the official work time of 40 hours.

Individual functions occupy the following percentages of official work time:

preventive care	19%
curative care	21%
health promotion	15%
supportive tasks	12%
management	9%
information tasks	6%
learning/teaching	12%
research	3%

Comments

In the light of the priorities assigned to the health centre's objectives, this represents a balanced allocation of time to the various functions.

Use of time is also efficient: only 1 h 10 min remains unaccounted for, and is probably unproductive time. This represents just 3% of official work time.

The allocation of time by the Public Health Nurse should be examined in the context of the health team as a whole; comparison with similar analyses for other staff members would make the results more informative.

Solution 54 (III.4) Preparing a timetable

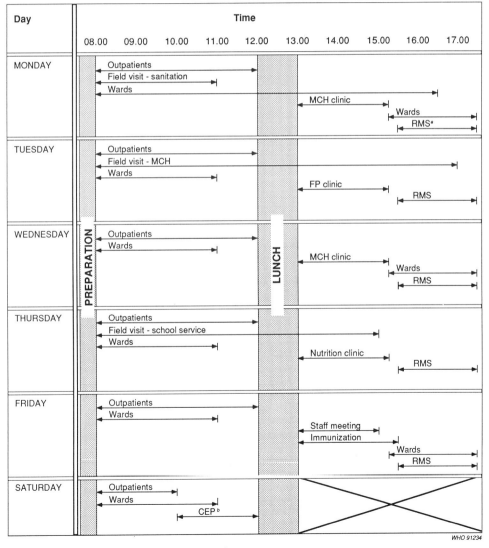

[a] RMS = Record-keeping, management and support tasks
[b] CEP = Continuing-education programme

Comments

Preparatory work is done in all duty areas between 07.30 and 08.00. Lunch-break is from 12.00 to 13.00.

Tea-breaks last 15 minutes; staff take staggered breaks between 09.30 and 10.30 and between 15.00 and 16.00.

The timetable indicates a balanced use of staff time. It shows that two main routine activities — outpatient consultations and ward rounds — take place every morning after the routine preparatory work. Field visits take place from Mondays to Thursdays, and continuing education on Saturday mornings.

Special clinics — maternal and child health, family planning, nutrition, and immunization — are held in the afternoons, and there are ward rounds on alternate afternoons. Completion and filing of records, and management and support tasks are carried out in the later part of every afternoon.

Solution 55 (III.4) Preparing schedules

Village	Day					
	Mon.	**Tue.**	**Wed.**	**Thu.**	**Fri.**	**Sat.**
A	Anna			Dora		
B		Bea			Ella	
C			Clea			Flicka

● Each of the villages is visited twice a week:

Village A — Monday and Thursday
Village B — Tuesday and Friday
Village C — Wednesday and Saturday

● Villages are always visited on the same days each week.

● Each nurse does home visiting only once a week.

Solution 56 (III.5) Managing work space I

Room X is used as follows:

07.30–08.00	Sterilization (a *staff* function)
08.00–12.00	Outpatient consulting room (for *patients'* needs)
13.00–14.00	Weekly staff meeting (a *staff* function)
14.00–16.00	Pre- and post-natal visits (for *patients'* needs)
16.00–17.00	Completion and filing of records (a *staff* function)

The following diagram shows the arrangement of Room X:

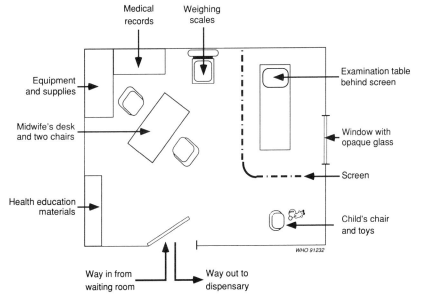

Area: 4.8m x 3.8m

Between 14.00 and 16.00 every day, Room X is in use for pre- and post-natal consultations. It is staffed by a midwife and auxiliary nurse-midwife, who see between 12 and 24 women at each session; about half the patients have one or two infants or young children with them. Thus there are between three and five people in Room X at any one time.

Considering in detail the facilities offered by Room X (where S – satisfactory, I = needing improvement):

Floor area:	18 m²	S
Walls:	Whitewashed 6 months earlier	S

Furniture:	Equipment, records accessible to midwife	S
	Chair for patient (or auxiliary nurse-midwife) and chair for midwife	S
	Child's chair is missing	I
	Examination table adequate	S
	(*but* paper towels are needed)	(I)
	Health education area adequate	S
	(*but* new chalkboard is needed)	(I)
	Children's corner lacks soft floor covering, toys and chamber pot	I
Access:	Entry, exit and movement within the room are easy	S
Hygiene:	Ventilation only through door from passageway	I
	Lighting, especially for examination of patients, is adequate	S
	The floor is soiled in places, needs scrubbing	I

For each room examined in this way, a table may be drawn up to summarize the improvements needed for the various activities that take place. The following is an example based on Room X above:

Improvements needed	Facility				
	Sterilization	**Out-patients**	**Meetings**	**Pre- and post-natal clinic**	**Records and filing**
Maintenance		Disposal of soiled materials	Cleaning of room	Cleaning of floor	
Furniture			Chairs needed	New chalk-board Child's chair	
Equipment	Basin and water tap			Soft mat, toys, chamber pot	
Access/ movement			Crowded to capacity		
Hygiene	Ventilation		Ventilation	Ventilation	
Other		Door sign: "No entry until called"			

Tables of this sort can be drawn up to summarize improvements necessary to meet staff needs, patients' needs, or — ideally — both. Any improvements that appear to meet the needs of both staff and patients should be given priority and implemented with minimum delay.

Thus, maintenance in Room X that improves facilities for both staff and patients, particularly as regards ventilation, would be given priority. The following table summarizes *who* should undertake the various aspects of needed maintenance and *when* improvements should be implemented:

Maintenance/ improvement tasks	Persons responsible		Timing
	for supervision	for execution	
Disposal of soiled materials	Medical officer	Assistant nurse-midwife Cleaner	07.00, 12.00, 16.00 daily
Floor cleaning	Midwife	Assistant nurse-midwife Cleaner	07.00, 12.00 16.00 daily
Purchase of chairs and chalkboard	Medical officer	Medical officer	When preparing next budget
Installation of water tap and washbasin	District health officer	Medical officer	As part of next structural change
Ventilation: — open window	Medical officer	Self	After each patient
— install ventilation channel	Midwife District health officer	Medical officer	As part of next structural change
— make space for staff meeting	Convenor	Secretary	As part of next structural change
Written sign on door	Public health nurse	Clerk	Immediately

Solution 57 (III.5) Managing work space II

The *staff* functions for Room X, identified in Exercise 56, were sterilization, record-keeping/filing and staff meetings. Assuming that the room is suitable for both sterilization and record-keeping, requirements for staff meetings should be the focus of discussion.

An average of 8 to 10 people meet once a week in Room X for 1 to 2 hours. By pushing the examination table and the screen into the corner, *space* is adequate for seating 8 people for the required time. However, staff must bring chairs from their own work rooms, since the two available chairs are adequate only for the convenor and the secretary. *Ventilation* is more of a problem for 8 to 10 people than it is for 3 to 5. *Lighting* is adequate if the screen is folded away.

Before meetings the *floor* should be *washed* (following the outpatient session) and all *containers* of soiled materials and used equipment disposed of; staff have objected to holding meetings in a messy consulting room and no alternative room is available in the health centre. Improvements needed should be recorded in the form of a table as in Exercise 56 and, after discussion in staff meetings, should be assigned as responsibilities to various members of the health team under the general heading "preparations for staff meetings".

Solution 58 (III.5) Managing hygiene in a health facility

The list of features where improvements in hygiene are required may be similar to the following:

Waiting room

1) floor needs sweeping
2) dusting required
3) sand in spittoon needs changing
4) through-ventilation is poor

Consulting room

5) floor needs cleaning
6) soiled materials need disposal
7) equipment should be stored after use
8) window should be opened between patients' appointments

Toilet

9) basin is clogged
10) toilet seat is soiled
11) walls are soiled
12) water tap is not functioning
13) swarms of flies

Corridors

14) floors and walls are dirty
15) rats and mice are seen occasionally

Incinerator

16) full of smelly unburnt refuse

Area around health centre

17) signs of indiscriminate urinating
18) waste paper

Wards

19) left-over food
20) soiled materials in corners
21) bed linen is soiled
22) ventilation is poor.

Unhygienic conditions may be a function of:

building design:	4 (partly), 22 (partly)
maintenance:	12, 13, 15
patients' behaviour:	9, 10, 11, 17, 18, 19
staff behaviour:	1, 2, 3, 4 (partly), 6, 7, 8, 16, 20, 21, 22 (partly)
work organization	most maintenance and staff-behaviour issues are to some extent related to work organization
resources	12, 16 — and, possibly, 9, 10, 11.

What can be done:

— to change patients' behaviour?	— health education while people wait — notice boards — public information — seek public support
— to change staff behaviour?	— recognition of problems — group discussion of alternative solutions — assignment of specific tasks and responsibilities — continuing-education opportunities
— to change work organization?	— staff meetings — supervision
— to improve maintenance?	— provide for maintenance in budget — regular site inspection — assign specific maintenance responsibilities — obtain public support for maintenance

— to improve building design?

— to improve resources?

— provide district health administration with information feedback

— provide in budget for expendable supplies and for durable equipment

Tasks should be identified, listed, discussed and assigned to individual staff at specified times or intervals.

Solution 59 (III.5) Work-flow arrangements I

The movements of 20 patients in health centre X were studied on one particular day. Ten of the patients were making first visits, seven were making return visits and three were seeking referral to the district hospital. Four patients were sent to the laboratory, to return afterwards to the consultation room. The times (in minutes) recorded for patients at the various stations were as shown in the following table, where the first figure is the shortest observed time, the second (underlined) figure is the mean time, and the third figure is the longest observed time.

Station	First visits			Return visits			Referrals		
Registration desk	3	4	7	1	2	3	4	6	8
Waiting room (first)	12	30	48	8	15	45	5	10	12
History-taking desk	4	6	10	Not applicable			4	7	15
Consultation room (first)	5	7	10	1	2	5	8	10	12
Laboratory	12	15	20	Not applicable			Not applicable		
Waiting room (second)	45	60	75	Not applicable			Not applicable		
Consultation room (second)	3	4	7	Not applicable			Not applicable		
Health-education room	10	15	20	Not applicable			Not applicable		
Dispensary	2	4	6	2	3	4	Not applicable		
Record room	1	2	3	1	2	3	Not applicable		

(Laboratory, Waiting room (second), Consultation room (second): for 4 patients)

From these figures, the following results were calculated:

	First visits		Return visits	Referrals
	With lab.	*Without lab.*	*visits*	
Average service time (= sum of all staff time)	57 min	38 min	9 min	23 min
Average waiting time	90 min	30 min	15 min	10 min

	First visits		*Return visits*	*Referrals*
	With lab.	*Without lab*		
Average patient-processing time (=service time + waiting time)	147 min	68 min	24 min	33 min
Shortest patient-processing time	97 min	37 min	13 min	21 min
Longest patient-processing time	206 min	104 min	60 min	47 min

For first visits, the service time (without laboratory tests) was 38 minutes and the waiting time — 30 minutes — almost as long. In the best cases, however, there was no waiting time. At worst, the patients waited almost 1 hour for 30 minutes' service.

For those patients needing laboratory tests, service time increased to an average of nearly 1 hour and waiting time to an average of almost $2\frac{1}{2}$ hours.

The analysis indicates that three particular points need attention — the service time involved in first visits, the waiting time associated with laboratory tests, and the fact that some patients have to wait 2–3 times as long as others. The group must be able to try out alternative uses of time and space, and changes in work-flow, to remove bottlenecks and improve efficiency.

Solution 60 (IV.1) Household health survey

Because of the nature of this exercise, no solution is indicated.

Solution 61 (IV.1) Priority health problems of communities

The table on page 450 may represent either an individual or a group solution.

When the exercise is done by a group, each member completes a separate table; the different responses are summed and the total number of points given to a particular health problem is divided by the number of people in the group.

Health Problems	High frequency	Long-term disability	High mortality	High cost of treatment	Easily prevented	National priority	Total points
Unwanted pregnancy	/		/		/	/	4
Diarrhoea	/		/		/		3
Complications of measles	/		/	/	/	/	5
Diabetes		/		/			2
Acute respiratory conditions	/		/	/			3
Eye infections	/			/	/	/	4
Low birth weight	/		/			/	3
Malnutrition	/	/	/		/	/	5

In the 'solution' above, top priority has been given to the complications of measles and to malnutrition, and lowest priority to diabetes. (In a group of eight people, measles and malnutrition were allocated 40 points and diabetes 16.)

Solution 62 (IV.1) Selecting a strategy

Action related to specific targets	Expected obstacles and resource limitations
(a) One antenatal visit by 100% of pregnant women = 2000 consultations at health centre	Lack of information about pregnancy Transport difficulties from village to health centre Antenatal visit not seen as useful
(b) Three antenatal visits to 50% of pregnant women = 3000 home visits	Insufficient home-visiting staff Official transport unavailable or unreliable Health worker unwelcome in absence of head of household
(c) Supervised home delivery for 1600 women	Time of delivery not known Lack of telephone communication Local TBAs not ready to cooperate
(d) Contraception practised in 1000 households	Inadequate technology (contraceptive pills or IUDs) Failure of logistic support Belief in the value of many children
(e) Nutritional education and demonstrations for 60% of pregnant women	Village health committees not active Transport difficulties Lack of funds for purchase of demonstration equipment

The most difficult obstacles to overcome are those to (a) — antenatal consultations at the health centre, (b) — three home antenatal visits, and (d) — contraception. It would therefore be best to focus on activities (c) and (e). To carry out these activities it will be necessary to:

- Enlist the support of the village health committees.
- Involve known TBAs with the village health committees.
- Organize the nutrition education programme *with* the village health committees and the TBAs; in this way it will also become possible to:
  — obtain up-to-date information on pregnancies
  — use local resources for demonstration equipment
  — make transport available (of staff to 'villages and of pregnancy/ delivery emergencies to health centre)
  — retrain TBAs in modern midwifery practices.
- Use the attendance of TBAs at deliveries to introduce and encourage other envisaged actions, such as *one* (to begin with) antenatal visit to pregnant women at home.

Solution 63 (IV.1) Scheduling primary health care activities

Activities required to implement the strategy outlined in Exercise 62 for ensuring supervised home delivery of 1600 mothers and nutritional education and demonstrations for 60% of pregnant women:

Enlist the support of village health committees:

1. Prepare a brief, precise presentation of what is to be proposed to the committees.
2. Arrange a series of meetings with all village health committees.
3. Meet with each village committee to present proposals and try to persuade it to:

   3.1 register local TBAs
   3.2 pay registered TBAs
   3.3 encourage TBAs to take refresher training.

Involve TBAs:

4. Meet with TBAs to persuade them to:

   4.1 register for, and participate in, refresher training

4.2 cooperate and participate in nutritional education programmes
4.3 monitor pregnancies in villages and report to health centre staff.

Organize nutrition education/demonstration programme:

5. Design a programme based on information about the problems, needs and resources of the women:

    5.1 decide on priorities by questioning local women and women's groups
    5.2 write out provisional learning objectives
    5.3 write an outline of education talk and questions to be asked of 'class' at first session
    5.4 prepare demonstrations to help women reach their learning objectives.

6. Plan and organize sessions in all villages with village health committees and with TBAs.
7. Arrange to obtain logistic and other support from the village health committee and TBAs (meeting place, equipment, publicity, etc.).

Retrain TBAs in 'modern' techniques of delivery:

8. Review TBA refresher training materials and TBA training needs.
9. Schedule refresher training course.
10. Arrange a systematic way for TBAs to notify cases to the health centre and to communicate with the centre for other purposes.
11. Conduct the refresher course.
12. Antenatal home visits.
13. Supervised home deliveries.
14. Nutrition education sessions.

Provide services to the women:

For each of the activities 1–14, a responsible staff member and some resource persons must be designated, and a timetable must be set for producing the desired result. A logical sequence should be established, for example for Activity 4:

Responsible staff member:	health centre midwife
Resource for registration:	health centre clerk
Resource for meetings with TBAs:	public health nurse
Resource for monitoring pregnancies:	health centre (statistical) clerk

Starting date	Completion date	Staff time required	
1-3-1993	30-5-1993	Midwife	10 hours
		Clerk	20 hours
		Public health nurse	5 hours

Total annual staff time	Midwife	TBAs
Activities 1–11 (first year only)	133 hours	1 000 hours
Activities 12–13 (each year)	240 hours	16 800 hours
Total	373 hours	17 800 hours
Proportion of available time	373/2000 = 0.186 = 18.6%	17 800/(2000 × 100) = 0.089 = 8.9%

Implementation of these activities is therefore feasible in terms of the staff time required.

Solution 64 (IV.1) Estimating costs

Activities		Principal resources required				
	Personnel	Transport	Equipment	Information and supplies	Funds (other than salaries)
1	×			×	
2	×	×			
3	×	×		×	
4	×			×	
5	×		×	×	
6	×	×			
7	×		×	×	×
8	×			×	×
9	×			×	
10	×			×	
11, 12, 13 and 14	×	×	×	×	×

To implement antenatal care and supervised home deliveries, the personnel resources required are the time of one midwife and 100 TBAs as shown in the following table:

Activity	Midwife (hours)	TBAs (hours)
1	4	—
2	1	—
3 (in 10 villages)	10×3	—
4 (100 TBAs in 10 villages)	10×2	100×2
5		
6 } (nutrition education)	—	—
7		
8	6	100×1
9	2	—
10	10×1	100×1
11 (3 × 2-hour sessions in 10 villages)	$10 \times 3 \times 2$	$100 \times 3 \times 2$
12 (antenatal home visits — 100%)	$10 \times 2 \times 12$ (months)	2000×2
13 (home delivery supervision — 80%)	—	1600×8
14 (nutrition education)	—	—

Solution 65 (IV.2) Coordinating

People The people involved in activities 1–8 are:
— midwife, TBAs, pregnant women (plus driver, storekeeper, etc.).

Things The 'things' involved in activities 1–8 are:
— delivery kits, equipment, supplies, transport vehicles, record forms (=information).

Places The places involved in the various activities are:
— the health centre (e.g. for activity 4)
— women's homes (for activities 1 and 2)
— village meeting places (e.g. for activities 3 and 5)

Time Certain activities must be completed before others can take place e.g. educational materials must be written (activity 4) before TBAs can be trained (activity 5).
Other activities can take place at the same time, such as:
— training, maintaining kits, and supervision visits (activities 5, 6 and 8)
— nutrition education and updating of family records (activities 3 and 7

The addition of one further activity — case-finding of pregnant women (before the 6th month of pregnancy) — seems necessary to the coordination of activities, so that:

— pregnant women are identified (people)
— household addresses are noted (places)
— time of delivery is anticipated (time).

This could be designated activity 0. One or two hours of enquiry per month should enable each TBA to identify one or two new pregnancies.

It would be useful for the activity schedule to make specific mention of *coordination meetings*, which could be held monthly at the health centre with each village represented by at least one TBA and a woman member of its health committee.

Coordination instruments	*Issued by/to*
Work schedule of the health centre	Medical officer or assistant to the health team
Individual work schedule	Each health worker to the medical officer (and for own use)
Duty roster	Chief nurse to staff nurses
Duty calendar for field visits	Supervisor to staff
Job description	Supervisor to staff

Solution 66 (IV.2) Monitoring work progress

Activity	Aspect of work to be monitored
0	Number of new pregnancies (of women who did not attend the antenatal clinic) discovered and reported
1	Are these women attending for antenatal examination?
2	Are all home deliveries supervised?
3	Have village health committees arranged convenient meeting places for nutrition education?
4	Is the educational material ready for the next session (or for all sessions)?
5	Are nutrition education sessions being held on schedule in each village?
6	Are kits being maintained for all TBAs?
7	Have family records been updated for the previous month?
8	Is each village supervised this month?
3, 5, 6	Was transport available when required last month?
and 8	Was there any supply breakdown?

Transport   Should be monitored by the midwife in charge of the programme.

Any transport failures should be noted in the midwife's diary.

The driver's log-book should be checked by the midwife at the end of each month.

Supplies   Should be checked by the health-centre clerk.
TBA requirements that have not been satisfied should be noted by the midwife in her supervision report.
The clerk should check stocks of supplies once a month.

Purpose   To report to the medical officer in charge.
To raise these matters at staff meetings.
To prompt administrative action as necessary.
To improve coordination of the programme.

Solution 67 (IV.2) Monitoring performance

The midwife's tasks in relation to the activities discussed in Exercises 65 and 66 are as follows:

● Service activities 0, 1, 2 and 3 (provided by TBAs):

— supervision
— support
— information.

● Development activities 4 and 5

— write educational materials
— assess TBAs' learning needs
— assist TBAs' learning
— assess TBAs' progress.

The performance norms that pertain to these tasks are as follows:

● Supervision
   — frequency norm   Each TBA should receive a supervision visit at least once a year.

● Support
   — efficiency norm   No item of equipment or supply should be missing from any TBA's delivery kit for more than one month.

● Information
   — completeness norm   Household files should be 100% up to date as of 1 January each year.

— correctness norm	No more than 5% of the information in household files should be incorrect.
● Writing educational materials	
— relevance norm	Educational materials should meet the most important needs of TBAs in their local situation.
— technical norm	Training should be in compliance with accepted standard procedures set by national authority.
— pedagogic norm	Learning objectives should be specified in such a way that their achievement can be measured or observed.
● Training TBAs	All TBAs should receive at least 10 hours' refresher training every year.
● Assessing TBAs' learning needs	Learning needs should be expressed as tasks to be performed and the corresponding skills, not merely as knowledge.
● Assessing TBAs' progress	
— frequency norm	At each supervision visit.
— personal norm	Discuss with TBAs individually.
— correctness norm	Recorded as discussed in TBAs' registration book.

Solution 68 (IV.2) Monitoring achievement

The following aspects of achievement should be monitored on a monthly basis:

Services delivered

Activity 0	New pregnancies discovered	target 125–175
Activity 1	Antenatal visits (before 6th month)	target 125–175
Activity 2	Supervised home deliveries	target 125–175

These activities should be monitored:

by village	target 13–18
for each TBA	target 1–2

in order to reveal differences in performance between villages and between TBAs — some performances will be better than expected and some worse.

Activity 3   Nutrition education sessions   target 10
                Number of women attending sessions   target 200

This activity should be monitored by village to identify possible differences in performance.

Outcome of improved services

Activity 0   Reduction in number of births occurring to women not known to have been pregnant (compared with births to known pregnant women)
Activity 1   Reduction in numbers of first antenatal visits taking place *after* 5th month of pregnancy and increased proportion of pregnant women attending *before* 6th month.
Activity 2   Reduction in numbers of unsupervised deliveries — and thus increasing proportion of supervised deliveries.
Activity 3   Increasing proportion of eligible women attending the *full* course of nutrition education sessions.

Impact of improved services on maternal and infant health

Activities 0,   For women who received adequate antenatal care compared with those who did not:
1, 2   — reduction in number and proportion of stillbirths
                — reduction in number and proportion of infant deaths
                — reduction in number and proportion of maternal deaths.
Activity 3   Reduction in number of cases of diarrhoea in infants.

Training of TBAs

Activity 5   Number of TBAs completing full training course of 10 hours

This should be monitored village by village.

Outcome of improved services

Services delivered by fully trained TBAs compared with those delivered by partly trained TBAs (see above).

Impact of improved services on maternal and infant health

Impact of services delivered by fully trained TBAs compared with those who are not fully trained (see above).

Who should monitor?	*How frequently?*	
TBAs	Monthly	Services delivered
Midwife	Monthly	Outcome obtained
TBAs	Weekly	Impact observed
Midwife	Quarterly	Training of TBAs

To whom should information be directed?

To midwife from TBAs, *or*
To midwife from village health committees from TBAs.

How is monitoring being performed?

Services delivered *are* monitored.
Outcome and impact of services *are not* being monitored.
Training *is* monitored.
Outcome and impact of training *are not* being monitored.

Why are outcome and impact not being monitored?

TBAs are mostly illiterate.
There is no form on which illiterate TBAs can record events.
So far there has been no literacy training for TBAs.
The village health committee has not yet appreciated the importance of this.

Solution 69 (IV.2) Controlling deficiencies

Activity	Deficiency found	Who should remedy	How to control deficiency
1	Only 75 of 125 eligible women attending ante-natal clinic	Midwife TBAs	Review plans and arrangements for increasing uptake of services. Was the target realistic? Try to determine reasons for failure to reach target and act accordingly. When necessary, arrange antenatal care in women's homes.
2	20 TBAs well below target	Midwife Village health committee	Find out why (e.g. TBAs too young, unpopular or inexperienced). Provide more support and supervision.
	No complications reported	District Health Officer, Medical Officer, Midwife	Find out why (e.g. record/report form not understood). Redesign form, retrain TBAs.
3	Women not attending nutrition education in 4 villages	Village health committee	Find out why. Advertise sessions, improve facilities, evaluate teaching/learning activities.
4	Writing behind schedule	Midwife	Find out why. Set aside more time for this.
5	TBAs not attending	Midwife	Find out why. Update educational materials.
6	Cost of supplies unknown	Clerk	Enquire.
7	Births (and birth weights) not reported	Village health committee	Find out why. Train committee secretary. Provide incentive for reporting vital events.
8	Supervision visits to 9 out of 10 villages	Midwife	Satisfactory — unless it is always the same village that remains unsupervised.

Generally, the staff member or officer responsible for monitoring should also be responsible for remedial action.

Solution 70 (IV.3) Supervision

Untrue statement	Concern	Action/help needed to remedy deficiency and concern
1) There is a weekly timetable	No	
2) Each member of the team has a written job description	Yes	a) Bring to supervisor's attention concern about lack of job descriptions b) Draft own version of job description c) Ask for a workshop session on job description
3) There is sufficient equipment	Yes	a) Demonstrate shortage to supervisor b) Put topic on agenda of staff meeting
4) The health goals and activities relate to public health needs	Yes	a) Suggest that supervisor discusses this with village health committee b) Help village health committee determine goals and related health activities
5) There are monthly statistical reports	Yes	a) Prepare own statistical report and send it to supervisor b) Ask for a staff meeting to discuss this topic c) Organize simple records and procedures

2a, 3a, 4a: *make use* of supervision visit to seek supervisor's help and to correct deficiencies

2b, 5a, 5c: *take initiative* in proposing concrete solution

2c, 3b, 5b: *discuss and resolve* problems in staff meetings or continuing-education sessions.

4b: *provide guidance* to village health committee

Solution 71 (IV.3) Supervision and problem-solving

In preparing the supervision visit the midwife:

— checks availability of the drugs concerned in health-centre stocks — *available*
— checks amounts supplied to the village pharmacy over the past six months — *regularly supplied*
— checks the state of the revolving fund — *balance up to date*.

During her supervision visit the midwife:

— visits the chairman of the village health committee to hear the complaint directly — *personal opinion*

— discusses the complaint with other committee members to obtain confirmation — *personal opinion*
— interviews the health worker in charge of the village pharmacy to get his viewpoint on the complaint — *personal opinion*
— verifies stock-books of the village pharmacy, in which drug issues to male and female patients are recorded — *male predominance confirmed*
— discusses indications for these drugs to find out whether health worker knows them — *inadequate knowledge of indications*
— reports to the village health committee on stocks, issues, and indications, and summarizes possible actions:
    — change of health worker in charge of village pharmacy
    — train the health worker who is in charge of the pharmacy
    — inform the public
— seeks agreement of the health committee on preferred remedial action — *decision*
— informs the pharmacy health worker (if not present at health committee meeting).

After the supervision visit the midwife:

— reports informally to the medical officer or assistant in charge of the health centre
— revises instructions to health workers in charge of village pharmacies
— arranges for a one-day refresher-training session with all community health workers on the proper dispensing of all village pharmacy drugs.

Solution 72 (IV.3) Evaluation

Table I shows no cases of neonatal tetanus in 1990 in Villages L to AA. This may be because:

— no cases occurred
— cases occurred but were not diagnosed
— cases were diagnosed but not registered.

Since many of these villages registered cases in subsequent years, the apparent discrepancy for 1990 was probably due to a failure to register cases that year.

The total numbers of cases for the years 1991–1994 were 11, 10, 9 and 8, which is what may be expected when a programme of tetanus control is implemented. Thus, the target of 7 or fewer cases in 1995 should be met.

The mean yearly incidence of neonatal tetanus in villages A to K from 1990 to 1994 is as follows:

A	B	C	D	E	F	G	H	I	J	K
1.0	0.4	0.6	0.4	0.6	0.2	0.8	0.2	0.6	1.0	0.6

Villages A, G and J have the highest mean yearly incidence figures. This may be because:

— there are more live births in these villages
— these villages have better means of diagnosing the disease
— better registration systems operate in these villages
— these villages are at greater risk than others.

To clarify the significance of these figures, mean yearly incidence *rates* based on the at-risk population (i.e. the number of live births) should be calculated. Using the figures provided for births during 1992 in villages A to K, incidence rates calculated per 1000 live births are as follows:

A	B	C	D	E	F	G	H	I	J	K
4	1.3	2.1	2.0	1.6	0.7	3.2	1.1	1.6	3.3	1.9

This shows that villages A, G and J have much higher incidence rates of neonatal tetanus than the other villages, as well as more cases diagnosed and registered. It may be that these villages are not properly covered by immunization or that the umbilical cord is still handled in the traditional way. However, another explanation may be that the other villages had cases that were not diagnosed or reported.

Comparing the incidence of neonatal tetanus in villages A to K with that in villages L to AA yields the following:

Year	Villages A–K		Villages L–AA	
	Number of cases	Incidence rate (per 1000 live births)	Number of cases	Incidence rate (per 1000 live births)
1990	13	4.1	?	
1991	8	2.5	3	0.8
1992	4	1.3	6	1.6
1993	3	0.9	6	1.6
1994	4	1.3	4	1.0

The *numbers* of cases in villages L to AA in 1992, 1993 and 1994 are higher than in villages A to K. However, when these numbers are related to the numbers of live births and incidence *rates* are compared, there is little difference between the two groups. The differences that are apparent for the years 1990 and 1991 are probably the result of undiagnosed or un-reported cases in Villages L to AA.

On the basis of these data, villages A, G, J, N, P and AA might be expected to have one case each of neonatal tetanus in 1995; this would represent an incidence rate of just over 1 per 1000 live births, compared with a probable zero in the other villages. With so few cases, it should be possible to discover why they occurred and to prevent further cases. These villages may need special attention with regard to antenatal care, immunization of pregnant women, health education about handling of the umbilical cord, and strict supervision of traditional birth attendants.

Solution 73 (IV.3) Evaluating work progress

A. Number of retrained TBAs: 9
    Number of practising TBAs: 42
    Percentage of practising TBAs retrained: 21.4%
    The overall retraining programme has therefore achieved its target.

    Retraining has been completed in two villages (L and R).
    Retraining is under way in seven villages (A, C, E, F, J, O and U).
    Retraining has yet to start in the remaining 18 villages.

    Immunization targets (60% coverage) have been met in nine villages (B, D, E, H, J, K, R, U and Y).
    With the exception of village J, all the villages with high incidence of neonatal tetanus are those with poor immunization coverage.

    There are 12 villages where communication targets have *not* been achieved (G, I, L, M, N, P, Q, S, T, W, X and AA).
    In seven of these villages one case of neonatal tetanus occurred, i.e. an average incidence rate of 1.95 per 1000 live births for all 12 villages.
    Five or more messages have been diffused in 15/27 villages = 55.6%.

B. In villages E, J and U, all three operational targets have been achieved; the same is true of village R.
    Assuming that targets will have been reached in all 27 villages by 1995, *five* or more villages should be expected to achieve their targets

each year. Work progress in 1991 has therefore not been fully satisfactory.

C. Immunization and diffusion of messages are satisfactory in villages
B, D, H, K and Y, but none of the TBAs (one in each village) has yet
been retrained. In 1992 there was one case (in village B) of neonatal
tetanus — an incidence rate of 0.9 per 1000 live births. It might be
concluded from this that the TBAs are doing a good job and do not
need retraining, but one case of tetanus is still one case too many.

In villages A, C, F and O, the only target not met in 1991 was that of
immunization coverage. However, only one case of neonatal tetanus
occurred (in village A) in 1992 — an incidence rate also of 0.9 per 1000
live births. It might even be concluded from this that 50% immunization coverage is sufficient.

The results for these two groups of villages are no different.

D. The 14 villages that have achieved none or only one of the operational targets are G, I, L, M, N, P, Q, S, T, V, W, X, Z and AA. These
villages recorded seven cases of neonatal tetanus in 1992 — an incidence rate of 1.95 per 1000 live births.

In villages E, J, R and U — discussed in Part B above — the tetanus
incidence rate in 1992 was 0.9 per 1000 births, and in the villages
considered in Part C the incidence rate was also 0.9 per 1000. Thus
there is a clear difference in incidence rates between those villages
that are well or fairly well covered and those that are poorly covered.

E. Staff member L has a greater target population to cover in more
villages (3950 pregnant women in 16 villages) than staff member A
(3300 pregnant women in 11 villages). Their results and achievements
are as follows:

	Staff member A Villages A–K	Staff member L Villages L–AA
Percentage of TBAs retrained	25%	18%
Percentage of pregnant women immunized	55%	38%
Percentage of village heads diffusing 5 or more messages	100%	37.5%

On the basis of this comparison, the performance of staff member A is
clearly superior to that of L. The poorer performance of staff member L

may be partly explained by the greater number of villages covered, by their smaller size or by some element of the population's behaviour. Other factors that might be considered are ease of communication (e.g. road conditions), distances to be travelled, the population's level of education and economic status, and whether or not the villages have health committees.

F. Differences in performance between staff members A and L might be explained by differing abilities in the areas of:

— management
— communication
— leadership.

To assess whether this is the case, the supervisor should:

— accompany each staff member on a field supervision visit
— observe each one's professional behaviour
— note each one's shortcomings
— discuss with each one any suggestions for improvement.

Glossary

The definitions included in this glossary are intended solely for use with this publication; they may not necessarily be applicable in another context.

Activity — A group of tasks with a common purpose.

Allocation — The assignment of a share of funds and other resources to a definite purpose, programme or activity.

Assignment — Distribution of tasks and responsibilities to staff (in a health team).

Assessment — Identification and analysis of factors that may explain evaluation findings.

Attitude — General tendency of an individual to act in a certain way under certain conditions.

Authority — The power or right to make decisions and to enforce them when necessary.

Budget — A detailed estimate of the cost of a programme during a specific period. The amount of funds at the disposal of a programme.

Capital expenditure — Funds expended on permanent or durable goods (e.g. buildings, equipment).

Checklist — A list of items to be checked one by one, to ensure that none is omitted.

Communication — The transmission of information from one individual or group, by any means, to another individual or group.

Community — Individuals and groups living and interacting within certain boundaries (e.g. physical, cultural).

Competence — The professional ability required to carry out a task. Competencies are clusters of knowledge, skills and attitudes necessary to the performance of a task or activity.

Constraint — Restriction or limitation of freedom. See *limitation* and *obstacle*.

Control — The process of verifying programme implementation, and of correcting factors that may prevent the programme from achieving its defined goals.

Coordination	The process of bringing the activities of different persons into relation with one another so as to achieve a common goal.
Cost	Resources expended in carrying out activities, including capital (or fixed) costs and recurrent (or operating) costs.
Coverage	Proportion of an eligible population receiving a stated service, or any service.
Criterion (plural: criteria)	Standard according to which something is judged or a decision is made.
Data	Elements of information, usually unprocessed.
Decision	A choice made between two or more alternatives.
Delegation (of authority)	The action of a person in entrusting authority, for a specific purpose, to another person.
Development	The economic growth of a society together with social improvements (for example, in health, education, and housing).
Discrepancy	A difference between what is found and what is expected.
Effectiveness	A measure of the degree of attainment of pre-determined objectives.
Efficiency	A measure of how economically resources are utilized to achieve predetermined objectives.
Evaluation	A judgement of value, based on observation or measurement or examination — for instance, the extent to which a programme has been effective and efficient.
Facilities	Buildings and equipment (such as health centres, hospitals, laboratories).
Feedback	The flow of information back from one stage in a cycle or process or system to a preceding stage, as a basis for further development.
Function	A group of activities with a common purpose.
Functional chart	A chart showing functions and lines of authority and communication within an organization. (Also called *organizational chart*.)

Goal	The intended end-result or achievement of a programme or activity.
Guidelines	Suggestions as to how to proceed in implementing planned activities.
Health problem	A departure from accepted norms in the health status of a community; sometimes also an underlying cause of such a departure.
Health services	A system of institutions, people, technologies and resources designed to improve the health status of a population. Also: the services provided to the population (e.g. preventive, promotional, curative, etc.).
Health status	The degree to which the health of a specified population meets accepted norms (of mortality, morbidity, impairment, etc.).
Health system	The set of factors (economic, social, cultural, political), including the health services, that determine the health status of a population at any time.
Implementation	Putting a programme into action; doing the work.
Incentive	Something that encourages a person to take action.
Incidence (rate)	The number of new cases (of a disease), as a proportion of the total population or of the population at risk, in a year or any given period.
Indicator	A measurable variable for indicating directly or indirectly changes in status, effectiveness, efficiency or work progress.
Information	Data processed for a purpose (e.g. decision-making).
Information system	A group of people, procedures, methods and perhaps machines and other equipment, for the collection, processing, storage, and retrieval of information.
Input	What goes into implementing an activity, i.e. people, information, resources, time.
Inventory	List of items.

Job description	A statement of activities and tasks assigned to a staff member. (See *post description.*)
Leadership	Art of influencing, guiding and managing effectively.
Learning objective	What a learner should be able to do after, and as a result of, the learning process, which he or she could not do before.
Limitation	A deficiency of a necessary resource (personnel, materials, money).
Management	"Getting things done". Management includes planning, organizing, directing, monitoring and control, supervision and evaluation.
Monitoring	Observing, measuring and recording the way activities are being implemented. Monitoring leads to control.
Motivation	A drive that impels an individual to make an effort and take action.
Needs	Felt needs: needs recognized by an individual or a community. Real needs: needs recognized as a result of a professional or technical survey.
Norm	Authoritative standard or model; the expected amount of work to be done; typical pattern of behaviour of a group. (See: *standard*).
Objective	The planned or intended result of a programme or activity.
Obstacle	A difficulty, other than a resource limitation, that hampers the implementation of an activity.
Organization	The pattern of responsibilities, accountability, authority and communication in a group of people pursuing a common goal.
Output	The product of an activity or programme. In health work the output is a health care service (e.g. immunization).
Performance	The actual output and quality of work performed.
Plan	A statement of goals, objectives and outputs, and a description of the courses of action and the resources necessary to achieve them.

Post description	A statement of functions, responsibilities, accountability and authority assigned to a person occupying a post; it includes a job description. (See *job description*.)
Primary health care	Essential health care, accessible at affordable cost to the community and the country, based on practical, scientifically sound and socially acceptable methods. It includes at least eight components: health education, proper nutrition, basic sanitation, maternal and child health care, immunization, control of common diseases and injuries, prevention of local endemic diseases, essential drugs.
Priority	A preferential rating that indicates importance or urgency, according to given criteria.
Profile	The qualities, capacities, and experience needed by a person to carry out a specific function.
Programme	A set of interrelated activities, in time sequence, and a statement of personnel and other resources required, directed towards achieving a stated goal or objective.
Progress	Actual implementation compared with scheduled implementation.
Qualification	Evidence of completed training or successful examination in relation to a job.
Resources	The means (personnel, materials, money) required for the implementation of a programme or activity.
Responsibility	A function, activity or task for which one is liable to account; a duty assigned to a staff member.
Role	The behaviour expected from someone in a particular status.
Sample	A subset of a population, representative of the total population, used for estimating some property or properties of the population as a whole.
Standard	An accepted criterion for judging performance: frequently qualitative. (See *norm, criterion*.)
Strategy	A broad approach to achieving goals, within which programmes may be formulated.

Supervision	A way of ensuring staff competence, effectiveness and efficiency, through observation, discussion, support and guidance.
Target	A statement of a measurable output related to a certain population and a certain time.
Task	Work to be performed within a certain time; an element of an activity.